Dietary Options for Cancer Survivors

Dietary Options
for
Cancer Survivors

A guide to research on foods,
food substances, herbals and dietary regimens
that may influence cancer

Edited by
Glen Weldon

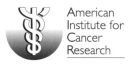

American
Institute for
Cancer
Research

Washington, DC

American Institute for Cancer Research
1759 R Street, NW
Washington, D.C. 20009
www.aicr.org

Printed and bound in the United States of America

ISBN: 0-9722522-0-7

Library of Congress Control Number: 2002109932

Contents

Research Review Committee

Acknowledgments

It took the application of many minds to produce a list we dare call current and almost complete. Matt Brignall, N.D.; Christina Chase, M.S., R.D.; Mark A. Mitchell; Beverly Westermeyer, M.L.S. and others all aided in the search. Melanie Polk, M.M.Sc., R.D. and Adrienne Forman, M.S., R.D. contributed to the introductory chapters.

Scott von Bergener designed the book. Ann O'Malley proofread it assiduously and more than once. Both saw it through production. Special thanks go to Kathy Ward and Jeff Prince of AICR, who after talking to cancer survivors and friends of the organization, conceived of this book and guided the project to completion. G.W.

Chapter One

Looking at the Research

At the American Institute for Cancer Research, we receive emails and telephone calls from cancer survivors every day. These people want to know what changes in their diet and activity level will help reduce the risk of secondary tumors or recurrence of their cancer. You can tell by their voices that this is a pressing question. They need guidance, and the health professionals they rely on are not offering it.

They are asking a reasonable question. They know that science has demonstrated an association between diet and risk of primary cancers. They conclude that adjustment of dietary intake can influence the progression of their disease, the development of a secondary tumor and recurrence as well.

They are probably correct, yet the scientific evidence to support this conclusion is promising but still incomplete. By way of illustration, consider the evidence supporting recommendations on diet and primary cancers. The expert panel that produced AICR's report, *Food, Nutrition and the Prevention of Cancer: a global perspective,* was able to cite at least 197 human studies that show a link between vegetables and fruit intake and reduced risk of first cancers.[1] They could have cited a larger number of laboratory studies that suggest how vegetables and fruits provide protection. On the basis of such strong evidence, they recommended a plant-based diet rich in vegetables and fruits as a means of reducing risk of primary cancer.

In regard to treatment of cancer and reducing risk of secondary tumors and recurrence, however, the evidence is nowhere near as consistent and convincing. Research is under way, but we have not yet seen enough congruent results from studies of varying design. In other words, the process by which science reaches even tentative conclusions is not yet complete. As a result, many health professionals are often reluctant to advise cancer survivors about diet and nutritional supplements.

Nevertheless, studies show that between 37 and 81 percent of cancer survivors use a variety of different foods and food substances as medicine.[2-4] Any number of reasons move them to do so. Some are simply determined to take advantage of every option to fight their disease. Others are concerned that their cancer will outpace the relatively slow scientific process. Still others may have reason to believe that none of the conventional treatments can help them and turn to alternative medicines and procedures out of desperation.

We have created this book for these people. Chapters three through six contain lists of all those diet-related interventions that might be of interest to cancer survivors. After every entry in each of the four lists, there is a summary of the scientific evidence concerning its effectiveness in impeding the progression of cancer, the development of secondary tumors or recurrence. These summaries are fully annotated so that people can read about the research results in the scientific journals in which they were originally reported.

These lists are comprehensive, not selective. In compiling them, we have attempted to include every diet-related intervention for which a serious claim has been made. Except in chapter two, where the general shape of a cancer-fighting diet is described, no specific recommendations have been made. The annotated lists and footnotes are presented so that survivors who intend to avail themselves of diet-related interventions can make informed choices.

If you assume that food is medicine, making thoughtful and informed choices about diet becomes extremely important. We know that the vitamins, minerals and phytochemicals in vegetables and fruits can reduce cancer risk. By the same token, research now suggests that some foods known to be cancer fighters – soy and beta-carotene, for example, – taken at the wrong time, in the wrong dosage or by the wrong people may actually foster tumor growth. Diets containing selenium seem to protect against cancer, but high doses are toxic, and the margin between safety and toxicity is narrow. Furthermore, some foods, herbs and supplements can interact with medicines, making these medicines less effective or too potent.

One graphic example needs to be emphasized. It is generally be-

lieved that antioxidants like vitamins C and E, beta-carotene and selenium are helpful in reducing cancer risk. But researchers have recently
raised a red flag about whether consumption of high doses of antioxidants during chemotherapy is helpful. Although some research supports
taking antioxidants during chemotherapy, other studies suggest they may
counter the effects of the therapy or enhance the growth of tumor
cells.[5-10] *Until more research clarifies this question, it is advisable for people
undergoing cancer treatment with chemotherapy or radiation to stop taking
dietary supplements with antioxidant properties for several weeks before and
during treatment unless advised by their radiation therapist or oncologist.*

All of this suggests that food and nutritional supplements have strong
effects on the body. That is why cancer survivors owe it to themselves
to learn all they can about the existing evidence before deciding on making
a diet change, taking a supplement or submitting to a diet-related treatment. Begin by consulting your oncologist or clinician. If he or she cannot
or will not advise you on dietary matters, consider finding one who will.
Diet is sufficiently important to the cancer survivor to warrant such a
change.

If you are unable to obtain the guidance you need from a qualified
health professional, you can use this book and other sources to investigate the existing research results for yourself.[11] When you have completed
a thorough study, discuss your findings with your oncologist or clinician. Show him or her your evidence and listen to his or her response.
Then you will be in a position to make an informed decision.

Several Kinds of Evidence

As soon as word is out about a cancer diagnosis, friends and relatives
begin to offer advice. They talk about miracle procedures, foods and
herbs that cured this aunt or that friend and insist they be tried. This is
called caring. It is also called anecdotal evidence, and anecdotal evidence in itself should be insufficient to make you put out money for
some special food substance or procedure and risk your health on it.

The trouble with anecdotal evidence is that it rests on one individual's
interpretation of his or her own experience. His or her circumstances
may be extraordinary; his or her judgment of cause and effect, too narrow. A patient who self-prescribes a supplement and then feels better
may well believe the supplement caused the improvement. In fact, any
number of other causes could be responsible for the happy outcome. It

is wise to remain skeptical about anecdotal evidence. Ordinarily, it takes a trained observer assessing the experience of thousands of individuals in controlled circumstances to reach valid medical conclusions.

Similarly, it is wise to be skeptical about the recommendations of a spokesperson or salesperson representing the producer, wholesaler or retailer of some food product or supplement. The object of any marketing effort is to sell the product. To that end, health claims that have little scientific foundation are often made. The language of a marketing claim often gives it away. The salesperson, advertisement or brochure will insist that the product can beat a variety of diseases – cancer, heart disease, stroke and many others. They will insist that the disease will be permanently eradicated – "we guarantee you'll be cancer-free." They will also use exaggerated phrases such as "medical miracle," "scientific breakthrough," or "potent, secret ingredient." Often they will offer unsubstantiated recommendations from individual consumers or health professionals without the proper credentials.

Even when marketers cite scientific studies, be cautious. Ascertain who paid for the research and who conducted it. Ask if it was reviewed by a panel of experts and where it was published. Studies that were sponsored by manufacturers or producers are not necessarily unreliable. Nevertheless, it would be wise to look for corroborating studies conducted by disinterested parties.

Don't let the recommendations of friends, relatives or commercial interests be the sole factor that induce you into changing your diet or taking a supplement. Ask questions. Look critically. The stakes are too high to act complacent. If the recommendation seems to have merit, do a little investigating. Look into the research yourself before taking any drastic steps regarding your health.

This book is organized so that you can see for yourself if the evidence exists to warrant your taking such an action. There are four chapters: Food and Food Substances, Vitamins and Minerals, Herbals, and Diet-related Regimens and Therapies. Look for the food, substance or treatment you are investigating in the appropriate chapter. Then, under that entry, you can read through a summary of relevant research results.

As you read, look for the characteristics that the experts value. When scientists review a body of research results, they tend to discount self-published reports. They look for reliable studies that have been peer-reviewed (reviewed by a panel of experts in the subject) and published in reputable journals. They assess the number and quality of the studies and look for replication of results. They also hope to find a sufficient number of different types of studies that confirm each other. (A discussion of the different types of studies and their strengths and limitations begins at the bottom of this page.)

In most instances, you won't find all of these characteristics in the research summaries that follow. It is hoped, however, that you will find a sufficient amount of consistent evidence to answer the following questions:

1. Have the benefits of this substance for cancer survivors been demonstrated?

2. What are the risks to my health in taking this substance?

3. How will this substance interact with the medicines I am taking?

4. What is a safe dosage for this substance?

If the science in the summaries does in fact allow you to answer these questions, you can make an informed choice. On the other hand, there may be too little reliable evidence reported or too little agreement among the studies cited. In that case, you should consider delaying your decision until more results are reported in peer-reviewed, scientific journals.

If, however, you choose to proceed without reliable science to guide you, you should at the very least learn all you possibly can about the risks involved. The following chapters include basic information on potential side effects and toxicity. A trusted health professional can provide a fuller picture tailored to your particular lifestyle and medical history.

Several Kinds of Research Studies

Why is it that cancer researchers look for agreement among a variety of different studies before they draw conclusions? Because there are many different kinds of studies used in investigating the prevention and treatment of cancer. Each has its limitations. None is perfect. Scientists believe that, considered in their totality, all the studies on a particular food or food substance will provide a comprehensive and nuanced picture of the truth.

Most cancer research is based on *epidemiological* studies. These studies of populations observe large groups – sometimes several thousands to hundreds of thousands of people – to see if there is a link between specific dietary or lifestyle behaviors and disease in a population. Epidemiological studies are observations of associations; they do not prove cause and effect. For example, they can identify a relationship between eating vegetables and fruits and lower risk of cancer. They cannot prove, however, that eating certain foods directly causes a lower cancer risk. People with a lower risk may have other healthy behaviors, like not drinking alcohol or not smoking, that offer them protection. However, when different types of epidemiological studies consistently show an association between a specific behavior and health outcome, like eating vegetables and fruits and lower cancer risk, they provide important evidence that a causal relationship may exist.

Common types of epidemiological study designs include ecological, case-control and cohort studies. Each has its strengths and limitations.

Ecological Studies

Ecological (or correlation) studies use large, diverse populations to compare disease rates, like cancer, with consumption of specific foods or nutrients. These studies are the simplest type of research for exploring the relationship between diet and cancer. They can generate hypotheses for more rigorous investigation, but they do not provide strong enough evidence by themselves to confirm a diet-disease connection.

Ecological studies generally use readily available vital statistics on disease rates, along with food disappearance data or data from national intake surveys to make their comparisons. But these studies are unable to control for confounding dietary and lifestyle factors that could explain the differences in occurrence of a disease. For example, some studies have shown a strong correlation between red meat and colon cancer. But diets high in meat are also high in fat and may be high in sugar and alcohol. Additionally, people who eat this way may lead more sedentary lives than people who consume diets with less meat. Without controlling for these variables, it is not possible to be certain that meat is the key factor affecting colon cancer risk.

Note that, to date, ecological studies have primarily been used to study rates of primary cancers broadly. To investigate recurrence and secondary cancers, smaller, more specific investigations like those outlined below are more likely to be used.

Case-Control Studies

Case-control (or retrospective) studies compare people with cancer (the cases) with similar people who don't have the disease (the controls). Researchers ask both groups what they typically ate in previous years to see if those with cancer ate more or less of some foods or nutrients than those without the disease.

Case-control studies can be done relatively quickly and inexpensively. Unlike ecological studies, they can eliminate or control for potential confounding factors. A major drawback, however, is that individuals may misreport what they ate in the past. Since they may be asked to remember back many years, there will inevitably be inaccuracies in what is reported. In addition, cases and controls may differ in how they recall their past diets, which could bias the comparison between the groups. For example, if people with colon cancer heard that eating plenty of vegetables and fruits protects them from the disease, they may report eating less of these foods because they developed cancer.

Cohort Studies

In cohort (or prospective or follow-up) studies, researchers collect dietary and medical information on a large group of healthy people (the cohort) and follow the group over time, usually for 10 years or more, to see who gets cancer. These studies can help demonstrate whether people who eat different amounts of a food or nutrient develop cancer at different rates.

Compared to other epidemiological study designs, cohort studies usually produce the most reliable information. Since dietary information can be collected before cancer develops, there's no potential for biased recall. The data may also be more accurate since the individuals are asked what they are presently eating rather than what they ate years ago. Additionally, cohort studies allow for repeated assessments of diet at regular intervals throughout the study and can examine the effects of diet on more than one disease at a time.

A major limitation of cohort studies is that they take a long time, since it can take many years for diseases like cancer to develop. Like case-control studies, cohort studies largely depend on their subjects' ability to accurately self-report food intake, which can give rise to certain biases. Additionally, with many thousands of participants needed to obtain meaningful results, collecting data and maintaining records on everyone involved over the years is expensive.

Most epidemiological research is observational, but it can also be experimental. Experimental studies include **controlled trials** and **basic research experiments** conducted with animals or in test tubes.

Controlled Trials

In controlled trials, people are randomly assigned to either an experimental (or intervention) group and given a treatment such as a vitamin that may affect cancer risk, or to a control group and given a placebo, or "dummy pill." The results of each group are compared to see if any differences between the groups can be attributed to the treatment. Not many controlled experiments are done in cancer research. It would be unethical to intentionally expose a group of people to something that could increase the risk of cancer. Controlled trials in humans are best justified when considerable evidence suggests probable benefits and no adverse response to the intervention.

The experimental method that provides the strongest evidence is a **randomized, double blind, placebo-controlled trial.** In such a trial, the participants are randomly assigned to either the intervention group or the control group. Neither they nor the researchers know who received the treatment and who didn't until the results are in. Trials that are blinded usually test the effects of dietary supplements in pill form, since it is nearly impossible to have a blinded trial with recognizable foods.

In randomized controlled trials, the researchers control the amount of nutrients or other dietary components that each group gets, which ensures a sizable difference in intake between the groups. There is also more control of confounding factors than is possible with the typical observational studies described above. Unfortunately, randomized controlled trials are expensive, and it may take a long time before differences between the groups can be identified. Furthermore, long-term dietary compliance may be a problem and the results of the study may not apply to everyone.

Basic Research Experiments

Basic research is conducted with laboratory animals (*in vivo* studies) or with cells, tissues and cell-free systems in an artificial environment like a test tube (*in vitro* studies). It adds support to epidemiological evidence and helps identify biological pathways by which dietary factors may affect the cancer process.

In laboratory studies, animals are used to test the effects of food and nutrition on cancer. They may be exposed to different amounts of nutrients or suspected cancer-causing agents, or fed various types of diets to see which dietary components increase or decrease cancer risk.

An advantage of animal studies is that laboratory conditions can be better controlled than can studies done on humans. Results of animal research may offer insights into the possible effects of a dietary component or food on human cancer risk, and may strengthen existing evidence by identifying biological mechanisms of action. But, laboratory animals are not little people. Due to differences in anatomy and physiology, findings from animal studies should not always be generalized to humans. Furthermore, to obtain significant results, animals are commonly exposed to levels of nutrients or carcinogens much greater than humans encounter.

In vitro studies of cells and tissues can help scientists identify cancer-causing substances and understand the effects of dietary components on cancer. They may help explain the mechanism, or how a biological process that causes cancer works and how diet can modify that process. *In vitro* studies add support to existing epidemiological research, but do not, on their own, provide good evidence on human cancer risk.

Finding Sufficient Evidence

When you have examined the totality of the research, you still may not find the kind of corroborating and supportive studies that will allow you to answer your questions about a food, supplement or treatment. If you decide to wait for more scientific evidence to be reported, remember that good science evolves slowly. New results may make great headlines, but they are probably not in themselves conclusive. You want to know how the latest diet and cancer study fits into the existing body of scientific evidence. Before acting on nutrition news reported in newspapers and magazines, on TV or the web, look for information that will place the study in its context.[12]

Whether reviewing the research summaries in this book or reading about research results in the media, there is one major principle to remember: Since each type of study is in itself incomplete, findings from a single study should not convince you to change your dietary intake.

The strongest evidence that a food, food substance or supplement affects cancer risk comes from different types of epidemiological studies, supported by experimental research and backed by identification of plausible biological mechanisms.

[1] World Cancer Research Fund and American Institute for Cancer Research, Food, nutrition and the prevention of cancer: a global perspective. American Institute for Cancer Research, 1997; 441.

[2] Sandler RS, Halabi S, Kaplan EB, et al. Use of vitamins, minerals, and nutritional supplements by participants in a chemoprevention trial. Cancer, 2001; 5:1040-5.

[3] Richardson MA, Sanders T, Palmer JL, et al. Complementary/alternative medicine use in a comprehensive cancer center and the implications for oncology. Journal of Clinical Oncology, 2000; 13:2505-14.

[4] Bernstein BJ, Grasso T, et al. Prevalence of complementary and alternative medicine use in cancer patients. Oncology, 2001; 15(10):1267-72.

[5] Lamson DW, Brignall MS, et al. Antioxidants in cancer therapy; their actions and interactions with oncologic therapies. Alternative Medical Reviews, 1999; 4:304-29.

[6] Prasad KN, Kumar A, Kochupillai V, Cole WC. High doses of multiple antioxidant vitamins: essential ingredients in improving the efficacy of standard cancer therapy. Journal of the American College of Nutrition, 1999; 18:13-25.

[7] Conklin KA. Dietary antioxidants during cancer therapy: impact on chemotherapeutic effectiveness and development of side effects. Nutrition and Cancer, 2000; 37:1-18.

[8] Prasad KN, Hernandez C, Edwards-Prasad J, Nelson J, Borus T, Robinson WA. High dose of multiple antioxidant vitamins: essential ingredients in improving the efficacy of standard cancer therapy. Journal of the American College of Nutrition, 1994; 17:13-25.

[9] Labriola D, Livingston R. Possible interactions between dietary antioxidants and chemotherapy. Oncology, 1999; 13:1003-8.

[10] Kong Q, Lillehei KO. Antioxidant inhibitors for cancer therapy. Medical Hypotheses, 1998; 51:405-409

[11] Salgonic RI, Albright CD, et al. Dietary antioxidant depletion: enhancement of brain tumor growth in transgenic mice. Carcinogenesis, 2000; 21:909.

[12] Several websites offer reliable, up-to-date information on supplements and the research about them that is currently available:
http://vm.cfsan.fda.gov/~dms/supplmnt.html

http://www.berkeleywellness.com/html/ds/dsSupplements.php

http://www.cc.nih.gov/ccc/supplements

http://www.nal.usda.gov/fnic/etext/000068.html

http://www.cancer.org

http://nccam.nih.gov/fcp/factsheets/index.html

http://navigator.tufts.edu/hottopics.html
This site evaluates the reliability of a variety of nutrition websites. Just click on "Vitamins and Minerals."

Chapter Two

Recommendations Concerning Diet and Exercise

A great deal of research has been completed in regard to diet (the usual pattern of food choices) and exercise (the usual level of activity) and their link to reduced cancer risk. In 1997, a landmark report was released by the American Institute for Cancer Research and the World Cancer Research Fund (WCRF UK) entitled *Food, Nutrition and the Prevention of Cancer: a global perspective*.[1] This report resulted from a review of more than 4,500 research studies on the relationship between diet and cancer and between exercise and cancer conducted around the world. An expert panel of 15 internationally known diet and cancer researchers conducted the review and composed the 650-page document. Their work has been translated into several languages and currently serves as the primary source for international dietary recommendations for cancer prevention.

The expert panel reviewed this large body of research in regard to the association between dietary choices and cancer at 18 sites and rated the evidence as "possible," "probable," or "convincing." It also reviewed research on the relation of exercise and body weight to cancer in 18 sites and rated it using the same terminology. After completing this review, the expert panel felt it had sufficient evidence to issue a series of recommendations for changes in diet and activity level that will reduce cancer risk.

In regard to these recommendations, there is one caveat for cancer survivors. Almost all the research reviewed focuses on reducing the risk of primary cancers. One might assume that substances that affect the first occurrences will also affect secondary tumors and recurrences, but that has not yet been demonstrated. AICR is actively promoting more research involving people who have been diagnosed with cancer. In the interim, most experts seem to agree that cancer survivors should consider research results regarding risk reduction for primary cancers as being relevant to their situation. Furthermore, most experts would agree that, except during treatment when intake of calories may be a more important consideration than source of calories, cancer survivors would profit from following the recommendations issued in *Food, Nutrition and the Prevention of Cancer.*

The recommendations have been grouped under seven headings to facilitate your relating them to daily choices about food and activity. The seven categories are plant-based foods, animal-based foods, fat, salt, alcohol, food preparation and energy balance.

PLANT-BASED FOODS

Primary Recommendation:
Choose predominantly plant-based diets rich in a variety of vegetables and fruits …

Related Recommendations:
Eat five or more servings a day of a variety of vegetables and fruits, all year round.

Eat more than seven servings a day of a variety of grains, beans, roots and tubers …

Prefer minimally processed foods …

Eating a mostly plant-based diet is considered by researchers to be essential to reducing cancer risk. Vegetables, fruits, whole grains and beans contain vitamins, minerals and natural substances called phytochemicals that help our bodies destroy carcinogens before they cause cancer. They can even help to stop or slow down the cancer process.

Research shows that just the simple change of eating at least five servings of vegetables and fruits per day could decrease cancer incidence by 20 percent.

According to the AICR report, there is a strong and consistent pattern showing that diets high in vegetables and fruits decrease the risk of many cancers, and perhaps cancer in general. At least 37 cohort, 196 case-control and 14 ecological studies have investigated the relationship between vegetable and fruit consumption and the risk of cancer. Of a total of 247 studies, 80 percent have shown a statistically protective association for cancers of the digestive tract. When studies of all cancer sites are examined together, 78 percent show a significant decrease in risk of cancer.[2]

Of all food items, vegetables and fruits are the most protective. There is "convincing" evidence that they protect people from cancers of the colon, stomach, rectum, esophagus, lung and pharynx. They "probably" also offer protection from cancers of the breast, bladder, pancreas and larynx. And they "possibly" also offer protection from cancers of the liver, ovary, uterus, cervix, prostate, thyroid and kidney.[3]

ANIMAL-BASED FOODS

If eaten at all, limit intake of red meat to less than three ounces daily.

Cancer-related research in regard to animal-based foods has generally focused on red meat and, more recently, on dairy products. (The role of fat, in general, as it relates to cancer is considered in the next section.) Poultry has not received much study in this regard, and fish has been studied for the protective effects of the omega-3 fatty acids it contains. (See page 27.)

The expert panel found, however, "probable" evidence that diets containing substantial amounts of red meat increase the risk of colon cancer. The risk of cancers of the pancreas, breast, prostate and kidney are also "possibly" increased.[4]

It is difficult to interpret much of the existing data as there are several possible reasons for this increase in risk. Diets high in meat are frequently high in calories as well as high in fat, both of which may be associated with increased cancer risk. In addition, methods of preparation and preservation may also play a role. (Cooking methods are discussed on page 17.) Preservation, such as curing and smoking, may increase cancer risk. Diets high in cured meats possibly increase the risk of colorectal cancer.

For colorectal cancer, 7 cohort studies and 26 case-control studies have examined the link to red meat. Two thirds of the more rigorous studies show an increased risk of this cancer with higher meat intake.[5]

The link between red meat and other cancers is only "possible," since limited research has been done.

Recently, attention has focused on the link between dairy products, or often more specifically milk, and prostate cancer. The expert panel report cites seven studies that show an association between milk and prostate cancer and four large cohort studies that show no association. It rates the evidence for a link as "possible."[6]

Since publication of the report, organizations representing vegetarian interests or the dairy industry have repeatedly made contradictory claims about the link between milk and prostate cancer. As a result, in 2002, AICR did a comprehensive analysis of the scientific literature relating to this topic.[7] Conducted by Dr. Helen Norman and Dr. Ritva Butrum, this review of the research suggests that the results of the human studies are conflicting and contradictory. Furthermore, although a plausible mechanism involving the interaction between calcium and vitamin D has been suggested, *in vitro* studies have failed so far to demonstrate that reducing the intake of calcium from milk would affect blood levels of the active form of vitamin D.

To date, the evidence is too inconsistent to warrant any recommendation concerning lowfat dairy products and cancer. But this is an area to be watched.

FAT

Limit consumption of fatty foods, particularly those of animal origin. Choose modest amounts of appropriate vegetable oils.

For many years, researchers believed that excessive dietary fat was a major factor affecting cancer risk. Recent research has caused experts to regard other factors as more important. Nevertheless, the expert panel concluded that diets high in total fat "possibly" increase the risk of cancers of the lung, colon, breast and prostate, and that diets high in animal fat and/or saturated fat "possibly" increase the risk of cancers of the lung, colon, breast, uterus and prostate.

It is possible that, as a general rule, diets high in fat may also be high in calories and therefore lead to obesity. There is "convincing" evidence that obesity increases the risk of uterine cancer and "probably" increases the risk of postmenopausal breast and kidney cancers.

In addition, diets that are high in fat may be low in fruits and vegetables and high in meat. The resulting lack of protective substances in the diet may in fact be a significant reason for an increased cancer risk in diets high in fat.

There are 11 cohort studies and 23 case-control studies that have examined total fat intake and the risk of breast cancer. Results are somewhat inconsistent, but indicate a possible increase in risk with higher intake, again, perhaps because of an increase of the risk of obesity and the resulting increase in risk of postmenopausal breast cancer. A total of 28 studies show that saturated fat can increase the risk of breast cancer.[8]

Current research seems to suggest that the type of dietary fat consumed is an important consideration for treatment of cardiovascular disease and possibly for cancer. There is some evidence suggesting that omega-3 fatty acids (found in flaxseed oil, canola oil, walnuts and fatty fish) may retard tumor growth, whereas omega-6 fatty acids (found in many vegetable oils, including corn oil, sunflower oil and safflower oil) may foster tumor development. A significant number of laboratory studies have examined the effects of these fatty acids on progression of cancer cells. They seem to influence cancer development indirectly by influencing the immune system. Researchers have had difficulty relating these animal and tissue studies to humans largely because the precise role of the immune system in human cancers is not known.[9]

SALT

Limit consumption of salted foods and use of cooking and table salt. Use herbs and spices to season foods.

According to the AICR report, diets high in salted foods and in table salt "probably" increase the risk of stomach cancer. One cohort study and sixteen case-control and one ecological study estimate overall sodium intake. Most report significant increases in the risk of stomach cancer with higher intake.[10]

Stomach cancer rates are generally highest in those parts of the world where diets traditionally are very salty because meat, fish, vegetables and other foods are preserved by salting. This includes Japan, parts of China and Latin America. Those populations which consume large amounts of salted fish have an increased risk of cancer of the nasopharynx. In general, this is not a concern in the United States. However, it is prudent to be aware of the salt content of foods.

Salt is used extensively by industry as a preservative and flavor enhancer. It is wise to read the Nutrition Facts label to determine whether a product is high in sodium, or to compare products to select one that is lower in sodium when possible. Moderation of sodium intake may be related to the risk of other health problems, including high blood pressure.

ALCOHOL

Limit alcoholic drinks to less than two drinks a day for men and one for women.

The AICR report shows a "convincing" relationship between alcohol consumption and cancers of the mouth and pharynx, larynx, esophagus and liver. In addition, alcohol is "probably" linked to cancers of the colon, rectum and breast, and "possibly" related to lung cancer. The link is greatly increased if drinkers also smoke. In general, risk is related to the amount of alcohol that is consumed, that is, the larger the number of drinks – and the longer the individual has been drinking heavily – the greater the cancer risk.

Most of the research on alcohol has been conducted on parts of the body that are directly in contact with alcohol. More than 21 cohort studies and 40 case-control studies show a direct relationship between alcohol and cancers of the mouth, pharynx and esophagus. "Convincing" evidence is also seen between alcohol and cancer of the larynx in 6 cohort and 17 case-control studies. For liver cancer, 19 case-control and 18 cohort studies show a strong relationship to alcohol. An increased risk of colon cancer is seen in 11 cohort studies and more than 20 case-control studies. Alcohol "probably" increases the risk of breast cancer, and this is clearly supported by 11 cohort and 36 case-control studies.[11]

Although there is increasing evidence that moderate alcohol consumption can decrease the risk of heart disease, it is clear that alcohol by itself may behave like a carcinogen. There are many other ways of decreasing the risk of heart disease such as losing weight, cutting down on saturated and total fat in the diet and increasing physical activity. Consider the level of risk of these diseases. For example, if there is a strong family history of cancer, you might want to be especially careful about alcohol consumption. If you are genetically predisposed to develop heart disease, however, small amounts of alcohol could be considered.

PREPARATION

Do not eat charred food…consume the following only occasionally: meat and fish grilled in direct flame, cured and smoked meats.

Grilling, broiling and barbecuing are considered to be high-heat methods of food preparation. These methods can lead to the formation of cancer causing substances. Polycyclic aromatic hydrocarbons (PAHs) and heterocyclic amines (HCAs) can form when fat drips onto hot coals and the direct flame is in contact with animal protein. The expert panel report concluded that diets high in meat cooked at high temperatures "possibly" increase the risk of stomach and colorectal cancers. A small number of epidemiological studies reviewing the frequency of consumption of grilled foods show an increase in stomach cancer cases.[12]

Although the evidence is not strong at this time, it is reasonable to exercise care when preparing foods to decrease the formation of carcinogenic substances. Marinating meats before cooking, flipping burgers and other meats frequently, removing all visible fat before grilling and microwaving meat for part of the cooking time all can help to significantly cut down on the production of cancer-causing substances. Remove any char that forms on food before eating. Substituting vegetables and fruits for some of the meat increases the total number of servings of produce in your daily diet and reduces exposure to charred meat.

When comparing the strength of evidence regarding cancer risk, it is clear that consumption of vegetables and fruits offers strong protection, whereas modification of cooking strategies for lower cancer risk may be useful, but not nearly as strongly supported by existing research.

ENERGY BALANCE

Avoid being … overweight and limit weight gain during adulthood …
…Take an hour's brisk walk or similar exercise daily …

According to the AICR report, energy imbalance (eating more calories than the body burns) leading to overweight and obesity increases the risk of some cancers. It is believed that there may be a number of other factors beyond calorie intake and physical activity behind this relationship. These other factors include type of physical activity, rate of childhood growth and age at puberty, fat intake and circulating insulin levels.

Currently, there is great interest in insulin and several related hormones (collectively known as "growth factors") that have been shown to speed up cell growth and division. When cell growth is speeded up, the chances increase that something could go wrong during the process, such as a random mutation that can lead to cancer. In overweight and obese individuals, tissues are exposed to high levels of insulin and other growth factors over an extended period of time, causing cells to reproduce continually at an increased rate. Colon cells, which reproduce quickly under normal circumstances, have been shown to be particularly susceptible to these effects. This may be one reason risk for colon cancer is higher in overweight and obese individuals.

The "insulin-resistance syndrome" seems to increase the risk of hormone related cancers (for example breast and prostate cancers) and colon cancer when chronic exposure to insulin stimulates the growth of cells. Physical activity may help to decrease levels of circulating insulin, and therefore may explain the decreased risk offered by regular exercise.

A recently completed AICR review of the literature indicates that numerous epidemiological studies have investigated the role of obesity in relation to cancer risk.[13] There is strong evidence for an association of obesity with the risk of post-menopausal breast cancer, and cancers of the colon, pancreas, uterus, prostate, kidney, ovary and, indirectly, esophagus. In addition, there is some consensus in the literature that overweight individuals experience an increased cancer risk, and that cancer risk generally increases as Body Mass Index (BMI) increases. A large prospective cohort study of non-smokers in the U.S. suggests that about 10 percent of all cancer deaths are caused by being overweight.[14]

Five case-control and six cohort studies show "convincing" evidence that obesity increases the risk of endometrial cancer. Most of nineteen case-control and three cohort studies show that there is "probably" a relationship between high body mass and post-menopausal breast cancer. Eight out of nine case-control studies show that obesity "probably" increases the risk of kidney cancer.[15]

More than 100 epidemiological studies have linked increasing physical activity to reducing cancer risk. There is "convincing" evidence that high levels of physical activity decrease the risk of colon cancer. High levels of exercise also "possibly" protect against breast cancer.[16] It is often difficult to interpret the effect of physical activity on cancer risk without considering how it interacts with other factors. For example, individuals who engage in regular exercise may also be more careful about their calorie intake and engage in healthier lifestyle habits, in general. They might eat more fruits and vegetables, not smoke and may be less likely to overeat. Therefore, it is important to examine many factors related to weight when considering risk of developing cancer.

[1] World Cancer Research Fund and American Institute for Cancer Research. Food, nutrition, and the prevention of cancer: a global perspective. American Institute for Cancer Research, 1997.

[2] Ibid., 441.

[3] Ibid., 437.

[4] Ibid., 453.

[5] Ibid., 455.

[6] Ibid., 461.

[7] Is milk a risk factor for prostate cancer? American Institute for Cancer Research, 2002.

[8] Food, nutrition, and the prevention of cancer. 390-2.

[9] Ibid., 269.

[10] Ibid., 492.

[11] Ibid., 401-3.

[12] Ibid., 500.

[13] Obesity and cancer risk. American Institute for Cancer Research, 2001.

[14] Calle EE, Thun MJ, et al. Body-mass index and mortality in a prospective cohort of U.S. adults. New England Journal of Medicine 1999; 341:1097-1105.

[15] Food, nutrition, and the prevention of cancer. 373

[16] Ibid., 373-4.

Chapter Three

Foods and Food-Derived Supplements

Plant foods contain natural substances called phytochemicals that have been shown to offer a range of health benefits. Although phytochemical supplements may not be harmful at doses that approximate the amounts found in foods, they are not a substitute for a diverse diet high in plant foods. When discussing foods and food-based supplements, two points must be kept in mind.

First, each food listed below contains many different potentially helpful phytochemicals – including substances not yet identified, and hence not yet available in supplement form. In many cases, the research on a particular group of foods has to date been limited to a specific phytochemical compound or compounds. Much of the work done with cruciferous vegetables, for example, has revolved around sulforaphane, which induces the body to produce cancer fighting proteins (see below.) But many cruciferous vegetables also contain lutein and zeaxanthin, which may have separate effects on cancer cells. Similarly, lycopene is a widely studied and widely known component of tomatoes. But lycopene occurs as part of a "red family" of related compounds, and the tomato also provides vitamin E and vitamin C. Some studies suggest that the family of compounds found in tomatoes inhibit cancer cell growth more effectively than lycopene alone.

Second, no single food or food-based supplement should be viewed as a magic bullet. For example, adding flaxseed or fish oil to a high-fat, high-calorie diet and sedentary lifestyle is likely to have much less effect than adding such substances to a healthier diet and active lifestyle. The information in the following chapters should be considered alongside the advice on diet and exercise in Chapter Two.

SOY

Soy foods include tofu, soymilk, soybeans, soynuts, miso (soy paste), tempeh, soy burgers and soynut butter. The main active ingredients in soy that appear to have anti-cancer effects are called isoflavones. There are three main isoflavones in soy: genistein, daidzein and glycitein. Soy is the only commonly consumed food that contains isoflavones, which seem to act as phytoestrogens (plant estrogens). Phytoestrogens mimic estrogen in some body tissues but can also counteract estrogen under certain conditions. Soy also contains several other plant chemicals (saponins, phenolic acids, phytic acid, phytosterols, and protein kinase inhibitor) that may have anti-cancer activity.[1]

Two main types of soy supplements are available: soy isoflavones and soy protein. Soy isoflavone supplements are usually sold as capsules or tablets. Soy protein supplements (often called isolated soy protein), which are usually sold as powder, liquid or bars, also contain isoflavones. Generally speaking, 10 grams of soy protein contain about 10 to 20 milligrams of isoflavones. Food manufacturers are also developing and promoting food products with added isoflavones. These food products with added isoflavones may or may not contain soy.[2,3]

Evidence:

Cancer Survivorship

Several *in vivo* and *in vitro* studies have supported the possibility that dietary soy intake inhibits the growth of metastatic secondary tumors as well as primary tumors.[4-11] A review of 26 animal studies found that 65% of these studies demonstrated a protective effect of soy from experimentally-induced carcinogenesis.[12]

Specifically, metastasis of rhabdomyosarcoma (a tumor arising from skeletal muscle) was inhibited in mice by feeding soy protein.[13] In one recent study on soy and bladder cancer, several different soy isoflavones seemed to work cooperatively to inhibit cancer cell growth and cause death of cancer cells (called apoptosis) in the laboratory. In this study, and in a subsequent study by the same authors, the mixture of soy isoflavones was shown to target bladder cancer cells and interfere with their growth.[14,15] Researchers have also found that genistein has inhibitory effects on the growth of cervical cancer cells *in vitro*.[16]

In addition, recent research suggests that the deficiency of methionine (an essential amino acid) in soy protein may generally inhibit tumor growth.[13] Diets high in soy protein have significantly reduced the size and number of chemically induced tumors in mice, as well as incidence of metastasis.[17] In a study involving lung cancer in mice, dietary genistein was found to inhibit metastasis and increase the lifespan of animal subjects, but daidzein had no significant effect.[18]

Another study was conducted to look for a link between soy intake and stomach cancer mortality in humans. Dietary data were collected from 6,000 randomly selected households in Japan between 1980 and 1985. Mortality statistics were analyzed in 1995. The results showed that in men, high soy protein intake was linked to low stomach cancer mortality.[19]

Most of the soy research that has been conducted to date, however, has focused on breast and prostate cancers.

Soy components such as genistein and biochanin A have been specifically shown to slow or stop the *in vitro* progression of many types of prostate cancer cells from the latent stage to the advanced stage.[20] Genistein has also been shown to be a potent inhibitor of breast cancer cells *in vitro*.[21] Biochanin A also has inhibitory effects in these cells but to a lesser degree than genistein.[22] Dietary soy protein has been shown to inhibit prostate tumor growth in mice, although in this particular study, mice fed diets high in rye bran experienced greater tumor inhibition than mice fed soy protein diets.

Cancer treatment studies have been planned in which soy would be used together with conventional cancer treatment to see if the addition of soy improved the patients' outcomes.[23] One *in vitro* study tested this idea in the laboratory with prostate cancer cells. The combination of genistein and radiation was more effective at inhibiting cancer cell growth than either radiation or genistein alone, suggesting that use of genistein with radiation may have potential in the treatment of localized prostate cancer.[24]

In a series of studies with rats, tamoxifen therapy seemed to inhibit mammary tumor progression more strongly when combined with diets high in miso.[25] Other studies in cell cultures have found that soy components potentially make breast, cervical, ovarian, head and neck cancer cells more sensitive to the effects of chemo- and radiotherapy.[26-28] Supplementation with soybeans and genistein has inhibited the metastasis of human mammary cancer in female rats.[4, 5] In a later study, however, a similar inhibitory effect was evident when genistein was added to mammary cell cultures but was not evident in rat models.[29]

A study of 18 patients with non-small cell lung cancer found that daily ingestion of vegetables with significant quantities of coumestrol, genistein, and daidzein led to improvement in survival times, objective responses and inhibition of disease progression. The median survival time in the treated group was 33.5 months, and the median survival time in an untreated group was 20 months.[30]

Special Note on Soy for Breast Cancer Survivors

Under certain conditions, soy and soy components have produced estrogen-like effects *in vivo* and *in vitro*.[31] If these effects were to occur in humans, they could theoretically prove harmful to breast cancer patients who might have micrometastases (cancer cells that have spread from the original tumor).

When two clinical studies found that soy isoflavones seemed to mimic specific effects of estrogen on breast tissue in women, [32,33] these findings occasioned some concern in the scientific community. The studies, however, were of short duration and did not measure cell proliferation, the traditional marker for breast cancer risk. Instead, they measured separate aspects of cellular biology – DNA synthesis and breast fluid secretion, respectively – whose associations to cancer risk are not as clearly defined.

More recent clinical studies of longer duration have shown that isoflavone supplements did not alter another marker for breast cancer risk, breast-tissue density in premenopausal women. No definite recommendations can be made about this controversial issue, but a recent scientific analysis of available data concluded that soy consumption *by adult women* "probably has little or no effect on either breast cancer risk or the survival of breast cancer patients."[25]

General Prevention Data

Several *in vivo* and *in vitro* studies have suggested that soy isoflavones may offer protective potential against prostate cancer. One study found that rats fed soy protein and isoflavones from age 2 to 24 months had a significantly lower rate of prostate cancer than rats fed a different diet.[34]

A large, prospective study was done to determine whether drinking soymilk affects prostate cancer risk. In 1976, a total of 12,395 Seventh-

Day Adventists began to provide dietary information, including how often they drank soymilk. After about 20 years, men who drank soymilk most often (more than once a day) had a 70% lower prostate cancer risk.[35] Another study found that consuming soy foods was linked to lower prostate cancer risk. This case-control study included 3,237 men of various ethnic backgrounds.[36]

Two studies found that soy had little or no effect on hormones that may be linked to prostate cancer risk. In one study involving Japanese men, 35 subjects were randomly assigned to either a control group or a group that drank about 340 milliliters (1.4 cups) of soymilk per day for 8 weeks. Blood levels of hormones (estrogens and androgens) were not different between the two groups with one exception: estrone concentrations were somewhat lower in the soy group.[37] Another study also looked at soy and hormone levels in men. The 42 healthy men followed two different diets for 4 weeks each. One diet included lean meat and the other included tofu as a meat substitute. Only a slight difference in hormone levels was observed.[38]

One study tested whether consuming soy can lower elevated prostate-specific antigen (PSA) levels in elderly men. High PSA levels are associated with prostate cancer. The 34 men drank beverages containing soy protein and isoflavones twice daily for 12 weeks. Their PSA levels did not change during the soy supplementation.[39] One recent study, however, found that 50 healthy subjects who received 50 mg of soy isoflavone two times a day for three weeks experienced an increase in antioxidant activity in prostate cells that could theoretically inhibit the formation of cancer.

Much research is also being done on soy and breast cancer. One animal study looked at estrogen metabolism in mice that consumed soy extract and two soy isoflavones, genistein and daidzein. All three of these isoflavone-rich diets caused changes in estrogen metabolism that have been linked to lower risk for mammary cancer.[40]

One human study showed that healthy premenopausal women who drank soymilk had reduced estrogen and progesterone levels. Lower levels of these hormones have been linked to reduced breast cancer risk.[41]

Research with animals and humans has shown that consuming soy *early in life* may protect against breast cancer later in life. Some studies suggest that regular soy consumption early in childhood may alter breast tissue structures so that they are resistant to cancer later in life.[42] A recent analysis of the literature on genistein suggested that exposure to soy foods containing genistein early in life may help protect Asian women from breast cancer.[43]

In one recent study, Chinese women were asked to remember and estimate how frequently they ate soyfoods during adolescence (ages 13 to 15). The study included 1,459 women with breast cancer and 1,556 women without cancer. The results showed that women who reported the highest soy intakes had half (51%) of the risk of breast cancer of women who reported the lowest soy intake. Women with intermediate soy intake had from 69% to 75% of the breast cancer risk of women with the lowest intake. The link between high adolescent soy intake and low breast cancer risk was consistent for each soy food studied and for both premenopausal and postmenopausal women.[44]

Another article was published about the same population of Chinese women. This article focused on the subjects' current soy intakes in adulthood. The results showed that women with the highest soy intakes had a 34% lower risk of breast cancer compared with women with the lowest soy intake. The reduction in risk was greater (56% reduction) for breast cancers that were positive for both estrogen and progesterone receptors than for other breast cancer types. The reduction in risk was also greater (54% reduction) among women who said their soy intake had not changed recently. For these women, a dose-response effect of soy was found. However, a dose-response effect was not found when the statistical analyses included all of the study subjects (women with a recent change in soy intake and women with no recent change).[45]

Dosage and Toxicity:

No dietary recommendations exist for soy foods, and no study to date has demonstrated an optimal dose per day.[46] A recent toxicity study with healthy men found no significant clinical toxicity for genistein even at doses higher than any previously administered to humans (16 mg/kg body weight).[47] One recent prostate cancer trial involved consumption of 2 servings of soy daily, which provides about 50 milligrams of isoflavones.[1]

Asian cultures are estimated to consume an average of 1 to 3 servings of soy per person per day, which corresponds to about 20 to 80 mg/day of isoflavones.[48]

FISH OILS

Fish oils, also called marine oils, can be obtained by eating fish or by taking supplements. In general, cold-water fish contain the most fish oils. Some of these types of fish are salmon, tuna, sardines, bluefish, ocean trout, herring and mackerel. These fish are sometimes called "fatty fish." The active ingredients in fish oils are the omega-3 (also called n-3) fatty acids, which are a specific type of polyunsaturated fatty acids. Two of the omega-3 fatty acids have been studied extensively; they are eicosapentaenoic acid (EPA) and docosahexaenoic acid (DHA).

Note: Another form of omega-3 fatty acid, called alpha-linolenic acid (ALA), is not found in fish oil but is found in flaxseed oil and (to a lesser degree) in many green, leafy vegetables. See the section on flaxseed in this chapter for research on ALA and cancer.

Evidence:

Cancer Survivorship

Several *in vitro* studies have shown that dietary omega-3 fatty acids inhibit the growth and proliferation of tumors in colorectal, mammary and prostate tissues.[49-53] Many of these same studies have shown that omega-6 fatty acids (found in corn, safflower and sunflower oils) enhance tumor growth and proliferation. In these cell cultures, as well as in animal models, the overall ratio of omega-3 fatty acids to omega-6 fatty acids seems to be more important to antitumor activity than the absolute amounts of omega-3 fatty acids alone.[50 55] A different study found that exposure to physiologic levels of eicosapentaenoic acid and gamma-linolenic acid increased the rate of destruction of prostate cells *in vitro*.[56]

One study evaluated the potential usefulness of fish oils for treating breast cancer that had been transplanted into mice. The mice were fed fish oil or corn oil during treatment with doxorubicin, a cancer chemotherapy drug. The fish oil increased the effectiveness of doxorubicin by slowing the growth of the tumors.[57]

In an *in vivo* study, mice were given diets containing either fish oil or soybean oil, along with the chemotherapy drug cisplatin. The fish oil diet inhibited tumor growth and metastasis, and thus had anti-cancer activity. Also, mice fed fish oil had no signs of cachexia (weakness and weight loss) or loss of appetite. Mice fed soybean oil did have anorexia and cachexia. Cisplatin with fish oil was effective against metastasis, but cisplatin with soybean oil was not effective.[58]

Another animal study found that diets high in omega-3 fatty acids in combination with chemotherapy increased the survival time of dogs with lymphoma.[59]

A study compared the recurrence of induced breast cancer in several groups of mice. Some groups began consuming diets high in omega-3 fatty acids 1 week before the primary tumor was removed, and the other groups began consuming high-omega-3 diets 1 week after the tumor was removed. Significant dose-dependent inhibitory effects were observed in the groups that began the omega-3 diet before surgery, but no statistically significant effects were observed in the groups that began omega-3 diets after surgery.[60]

In another study, however, omega-3 fatty acids promoted the spread of colon carcinoma in the liver tissue of rats.[61] A later study also showed omega-3 fatty acids to increase the growth and proliferation of tumors in mice.[62] Another study found that combining docosahexaenoic acid with the chemotherapeutic agent paclitaxel increases the rate of lung cancer cell destruction in mice.[63] The researchers found that this combination stayed in the target cells for longer periods than paclitaxel alone. The levels of docosahexaenoic acid in fat tissue have been found to be an important indicator of how tumors will respond to therapy.[64]

In one 1994 clinical study with 120 breast cancer patients, a high level of omega-3 fatty acids in fat tissue before surgery was associated with lower occurrence of metastasis, suggesting that omega-3 fatty acids may exert a protective effect in humans.[65]

Recently several clinical studies with cancer patients have investigated the effects of omega-3 fatty acids on the compromised immune system. In one study involving 20 cancer patients with solid tumors, fish oil supplements were found to increase T-cell and natural killer cell ratios.[66] In several other clinical studies, dietary fish oil has been associated with helping to prevent weight loss and boosting the immune system in several ways, reducing side-effects of certain treatments and, in some cases, prolonging survival time.[67-71]

In a recent retrospective analysis of a group of 405 brain cancer patients, a combination of radiotherapy and omega-3 fatty acids/bioflavonoid supplementation was associated with increased survival time.[72]

General Prevention Data

One study looked at fish consumption and risk of prostate cancer. A population of 6,272 Swedish men was followed for 30 years. The men who never ate fish had a rate of prostate cancer that was 2 to 3 times that of men who ate moderate or high quantities of fish. The authors concluded that fish consumption could be linked to lower prostate cancer risk.[73]

Many studies have found that omega-3 fatty acids have anti-cancer effects. In one study, EPA and DHA were fed to mice that were genetically programmed to develop intestinal tumors. Mice fed EPA developed only half as many tumors in the colon and small intestine as did mice not given EPA. Mice fed DHA had a less dramatic reduction in the number of tumors that developed. The results show that consuming EPA reduces intestinal tumors in mice.[74]

High-fat diets have been linked to breast cancer in some studies but not in others. Recent animal and human studies have provided evidence that different types of fat may have opposite effects on cancer risk. High intakes of omega-6 polyunsaturated fatty acids appear to promote colon cancer, breast cancer and possibly prostate cancer. In contrast, omega-3 fatty acids from fish oils appear to prevent these cancers.[75]

Dosage and Toxicity:

At this time, there are no absolute recommendations about a dosage of fish oil that might be most helpful for cancer prevention.

Fish oil supplements are often used for other medical reasons, such as treating high blood pressure, high blood triglycerides, rheumatoid arthritis, Crohn's disease and colitis. Typical doses for these conditions range from 1 gram to 5 grams of combined EPA and DHA daily. The 1 to 5 grams refer to the weight of the EPA plus DHA within the fish oil, but the weight of the capsule is usually much higher.[76] However, in one study conducted with terminal cancer patients, the maximum dose that could be tolerated without gastrointestinal complaint (diarrhea) was found to be 0.3 g/kg per day.[77]

Hemophiliacs, people about to undergo surgery and people taking warfarin (Coumadin) should note that fish oil supplements can reduce blood clotting and promote bleeding. Fish oil supplements can interact with other drugs and supplements that can affect blood clotting, such as aspirin, nonsteroidal anti-inflammatory drugs (NSAIDS), flax, garlic and ginkgo. Diabetics should be aware that fish oil supplements can affect blood sugar control.

FLAXSEED

Description:

Flaxseed is rich in substances called lignans. Lignans are in the category of substances called phytoestrogens (plant estrogens). These phytoestrogens may help prevent certain cancers.[78] Flaxseed is the best source of lignans in human diets.[79] However, lignans are also found in many other high-fiber foods such as grains, nuts and beans.

Flaxseed is sold as flaxseed flour, flaxseed meal (the texture of cornmeal), flaxseed oil and whole flaxseeds. The whole seeds cannot be digested, so they provide no nutritional or health benefits unless they are ground. They can be ground in a food processor or coffee grinder to make flaxseed flour or meal. Flaxseed oil does not contain lignans, but some manufacturers add them. Flaxseed oil is also called edible linseed oil.

In addition to being a rich source of lignans, flax is also high in an omega-3 fatty acid called alpha-linolenic acid (ALA.) Other forms of omega-3 fatty acids are found in many kinds of fish and several other foods (see above.) Omega-3 fatty acids, also called n-3 polyunsaturated fatty acids (PUFAs), are being studied for possible beneficial health effects, including cancer prevention and cholesterol-lowering effects.

Evidence:

Cancer Survivorship

Dietary supplementation with whole flaxseed and with lignans have shown a variety of effects that are believed to inhibit the initiation and promotion of cancers in cellular, tissue and animal studies. [1, 65, 79-90] Several possible mechanisms have been suggested to explain how flaxseed may affect cancer.[91]

Recent studies have indicated that flaxseed also reduces metastasis and inhibits the growth of metastatic secondary tumors. In one study, lignans was found to inhibit skin tumors in mice at two stages of the cancer process.[92] In another study, adding flaxseed to the diet of mice with skin tumors caused a dose-dependent decrease in tumor size and number.[93]

In one *in vitro* study, a combination of tamoxifen and lignans from flaxseed inhibited early-stage tumor metastasis in estrogen-negative breast cells. This effect was slightly stronger than the effect of tamoxifen alone. A different study found that the combination of alpha-linolenic acid with paclitaxel, a commonly-used chemotherapeutic drug, increased the ability of paclitaxel to kill breast cancer cells *in vitro.*[94]

However, the laboratory data suggest that many factors affect the anti-cancer potential of flaxseed and lignans. One study with mammary cancer in rats found dietary flaxseed to be more effective against early stages of the cancer process, while flaxseed oil was most effective on established tumors.[95] Another study found that while flaxseed did not exhibit a dose-dependent effect upon the progression of mammary tumors in rats, the general presence of flaxseed in the diet did appear to delay tumor growth.[96] Another study showed that the anti-cancer potential of flaxseed varies widely depending upon conditions such as flaxseed variety and harvest conditions.[97]

In a short-term clinical study, first-time breast cancer patients underwent a breast tissue biopsy and were then divided into two groups, one of which received daily muffins containing 25 grams of flaxseed and one that received control muffins. When the subjects were again biopsied 39 days later, those in the flaxseed muffin group experienced an overall 30 percent reduction in tumor growth.[65]

Note: To date, the laboratory and clinical work on flaxseed and breast cancer has focused on estrogen-receptor negative breast cancers. The effect of flaxseed and lignans on estrogen-receptor positive breast cancers has not been studied.

A recent clinical study measured the effects of flaxseed supplementation and a low-fat diet in men with prostate cancer. The 25 men were waiting for prostate surgery while they followed the diet for approximately 1 month. The diet was very low in fat (20% of calories) and included 30 grams of flaxseed daily. Various indicators of prostate cancer biology and hormone levels were measured before and after the diet. After 5 weeks, subjects on the flaxseed diet had more slowly-dividing tumor cells and a greater rate of tumor cell death than men who did not consume flaxseed. The results suggested that the flaxseed-supplemented, low-fat diet influenced several aspects of prostate cancer biology.[84]

General Prevention Data

In several animal studies and cell studies, flaxseed had effects that may protect against cancer.[79] For example, in experiments with rodents, flaxseed prevented tumors of the colon, mammary gland and lung.[1]

One study found that female rats whose mothers ate flaxseed during pregnancy and lactation had changes in mammary gland development that could be linked to lower risk of mammary cancer.[80]

In another study, however, mother rats were fed flaxseed which seemed to produce hormonal changes in their offspring (both male and female) that in turn altered the offsprings' normal development in ways that warrant further study.[86] Still other studies have shown that rats who consume flaxseed while breast-feeding may lower breast cancer risk in female offspring.[80] Recently, a biological pathway was proposed that appears to explain, at least in part, how flaxseed may exert anti-cancer effects.[81]

In some human studies, flaxseed had beneficial effects that may be linked to cancer prevention. For instance, in healthy premenopausal women, consuming flaxseed powder caused several changes in hormone levels that have been linked to lower breast cancer risk.[82] Another study of breast cancer risk in premenopausal women tested the effects of flaxseed and wheat bran supplements. Sixteen women consumed their usual diets plus the supplements. Estrogen metabolism, which appears to be a biomarker (indicator) of breast cancer risk, was examined. During the flaxseed supplementation, estrogen metabolism changed in a way that may protect against breast cancer. Wheat bran did not have this effect.[83]

A study about breast cancer risk in postmenopausal women also tested the effects of flaxseed. The 28 women consumed their usual diets with and without supplements of ground flaxseed. The authors concluded that the results suggested flaxseed may protect against breast cancer in postmenopausal women.[79]

The role of the omega-3 fatty acid found in flaxseed on the risk of first prostate cancers, however, is less certain. In 6 different epidemiological studies, high blood levels and/or high intakes of ALA have been associated with large increases in prostate cancer risk. Two separate and more recent epidemiological investigations, however, have found high intake of ALA to be associated with lower risk of prostate cancer. Another study found no link between high ALA intake and the growth rate of prostate cancer in humans.[98]

Dosage and Toxicity:

There are no reports of flaxseed oil overdosage.[87] Subjects in short-term clinical trials studying prostate cancer consumed 30 grams of flaxseed daily with no apparent ill effects. Subjects in a short-term breast cancer clinical trial consumed 25 grams of flaxseed daily. There is some evidence that the widely studied anti-cancer effects associated with flaxseed level off at doses higher than 25 grams.[65]

Hemophiliacs, people about to have surgery and individuals taking warfarin (Coumadin), aspirin, or nonsteroidal anti-inflammatory drugs (NSAIDS) should note that flaxseed and flaxseed oil may reduce blood clotting and promote bleeding.

Flaxseed may interact with other supplements that affect blood clotting, such as fish oil. Garlic and ginkgo may also interact with flaxseed.

TEA

Since ancient times, tea has been used as a beverage and also as a medicine. In recent years, scientists have collected much information about the active ingredients in tea and their possible health effects. Black tea and green tea are the two main types of tea being studied. Both types of tea contain numerous active ingredients, including polyphenols and flavonoids, which are potent antioxidants. Polyphenols are thought to have broad anti-cancer effects. Within the category of flavonoids, catechins are a type of very active flavonoids. Tea is the best source of catechins in human diets. Green tea contains about three times the quantity of catechins found in black tea.[99,100]

Supplements of green tea catechins and green tea extracts are available. These supplements are packaged as capsules, tablets, powder or liquid. Typical doses of catechins range from 125 to 250 milligrams daily. Supplement labels may list the specific catechins in green tea. The four major catechins in green tea are epigallocatechin gallate (EGCG), epigallocatechin (EGC), epicatechin gallate (ECG), and epicatechin (EC). Catechins are flavonoids and also polyphenols, and these terms may be listed on supplement labels.

Evidence:
Cancer Survivorship

Green tea extracts have inhibited the growth of leukemic and breast cancer cells *in vitro* and skin tumors in animal subjects.[101-103] In one study, catechins were mixed with cells in the laboratory. The catechins inhibited cancer development at all three major stages (initiation, promotion, and progression of cancer). Similar results were obtained using catechins to inhibit the growth of cancerous human colon and liver cells.[104] Catechins achieved these beneficial effects by influencing many different metabolic pathways in cells.[99] One of the ways that cancer inhibition is achieved is through apoptosis.

Still other research, including studies performed with cells in the laboratory, found that polyphenols in green and black tea appear to inhibit tumor growth and trigger tumor death.[105,106]

In a recent series of studies with mice, a diet featuring both green tea and soy protein was found to slow the progression of induced prostate tumors significantly more than diets featuring either green tea or soy alone.[107] Rats who consumed water containing 2% green tea developed lung cancer at a rate of only 16% compared to 46% in those that consumed water with no green tea. These animals were subjected to experimentally-induced lung cancer through asbestos and benzo(a)pyrene injections.

An additional study in rats found that dietary supplementation with 1% green tea catechins led to the regression of liver cancer cell formation.[108] Human prostate and breast cancer cells transplanted into mice were found to undergo growth inhibition and regression after exposure to epigallocatechin, a significant component of green tea.[109]

A Phase I/II study found that persons who drank green tea solids dissolved in warm water had short-term reductions in prostaglandin E2 levels in rectal tissue.[110] Prostaglandin E2 levels are believed to be an important factor in the development of cancerous cells.

In a large, recent follow-up study involving 472 Japanese women, subjects who drank 5 or more cups of green tea daily had reduced recurrence of stage I and II breast cancer after seven years. No improvement in prognosis was observed for individuals with stage III breast cancer, however.[111]

A similarly designed study involving 1,160 breast cancer patients found that consumption of three or more cups of green tea daily was associated with significantly reduced recurrence of stage I breast cancer after seven years. The effect of tea consumption on stage II recurrence was smaller, and did not affect the recurrence of more advanced breast cancers.[112]

General Prevention Data

In cellular and animal models, administration of tea and tea components have prevented several types of cancer, including cancers of the lung, skin and digestive tract.[99,113,114]

Human cohort studies found evidence that green tea may lower the risk for bladder, colon, stomach, pancreatic and esophageal cancers.[1,99]

The strongest evidence from human studies was found with green tea in Asian populations.[115]

Several studies of similar design and scope have reported no link between tea consumption and cancer incidence.[116]

Dosage and Toxicity:

No reports of overdosage from dietary sources have been reported. The way that tea is prepared, including the length of time it is steeped, may influence its anti-cancer potential. There is some concern that consumption of tea at extremely high temperatures may possibly increase the risk of cancer of the upper digestive tract.

Overdosage of green tea supplements has not been reported, but they have been shown to interact with drugs that affect blood clotting, such as aspirin and warfarin (Coumadin).[117]

CRUCIFEROUS VEGETABLES

The cruciferous vegetables, also known as brassica vegetables, are broccoli, cauliflower, cabbage, Brussels sprouts, bok choy and kale. This family of vegetables contains many phytochemicals (natural plant chemicals) that may help prevent cancer. These potentially beneficial phytochemicals include glucosinolates, crambene, indole-3-carbinol and isothiocyanates (which are in turn derived from other compounds called glucosinolates).

Available supplements include extracts of broccoli, cabbage and kale, and consumers should note that labels may not reveal the amounts of these vegetable extracts or the quantities of active ingredients contained in these extracts.

Evidence:

Cancer Survivorship

Much evidence has accumulated to support the theory that consumption of cruciferous vegetables helps prevent first cancers (see below.) These studies suggest that compounds in these foods regulate a complex enzymatic system that helps the body defend itself from the kind of damage that can initiate the cancer process. Recently, an increasing amount of data has suggested that these foods – and their components – may play a role in inhibiting cancer growth and tumor formation as well. High-selenium broccoli has been shown to inhibit both mammary and colon cancer tumors in similar animal models.[118]

Indole-3-carbinol (I3C) is a compound that the body produces when cruciferous vegetables are consumed, and this substance, along with metabolites such as diindolymethane (DIM), have shown the ability to inhibit the growth of tumors in several cell and tissue cultures, including those of the breast, endometrium, lung, colon and liver.[47] In one recent study involving a two-stage mouse/skin cancer model, indole-3-carbinol was found to reduce the number and size of tumors, as well as lengthen the amount of time it took for tumors to form.[119] I3C has been found to increase the 2/16-hydroxyesterone ratio, which has been found to lower the risk of developing breast cancer in many studies.[120]

In a 14-day clinical study, 29 subjects at high risk for colon cancer were randomized into two groups. Group 1 consumed no cruciferous vegetables, Group 2 consumed broccoli supplements (I3C) three times per day. This study identified specific changes in the blood of the two groups that will be used in future studies involving patients with a history of colon cancer.[121]

In a small study involving 18 juvenile patients with respiratory papillomatosis who were followed for 15 months, 6 patients showed no response to supplementation with indole-3-carbinol, 6 patients showed a modest reduction in papilloma growth rate, and 6 patients had a complete cessation of papilloma growth.[122]

A 12-week placebo-controlled study of 30 women with precancerous cervical dysplasia found that 200 to 400 mg/day of I3C led to significant regressions of disease compared with placebo.[123]

General Prevention Data

Many studies have shown that high intakes of cruciferous vegetables are linked to a reduced risk of cancer in general. The strongest evidence that cruciferous vegetables protect against cancer was reported for lung, stomach and colorectal cancers. The evidence of protection was less consistent for ovarian, endometrial and prostate cancers.[124]

One recent study looked at diet and prostate cancer risk in men of different ethnic backgrounds. Dietary information was collected from 1,618 control subjects without cancer and 1,619 men with prostate cancer. The scientists calculated that the odds of developing prostate cancer are 39% lower in men who eat the most cruciferous vegetables, compared with men who eat the least.[36]

A study of diet and bladder cancer risk found that men with the highest intakes of cruciferous vegetables had only half the risk (49%) of developing bladder cancer, compared with men who ate the least cruciferous vegetables. There were 252 cases of bladder cancer among 47,909 men who were followed for 10 years. The evidence of protection was strongest for broccoli and cabbage.[125]

Dosage and Toxicity:
No reports of overdosage have been documented.

GARLIC AND OTHER ONION-FAMILY (ALLIUM) VEGETABLES

The Allium, or onion-family, vegetables include onions, garlic, scallions, leeks and chives. These vegetables contain many active ingredients that may have anti-cancer effects. Some of these active ingredients (and the compounds they produce in chemical reactions) include allicin, allixin, allyl sulfides and quercetin. Allium vegetables are rich in organosulfur compounds, which appear to have anti-cancer effects. Onions are especially rich in quercetin (a flavonol, in the category of substances called flavonoids), which also may help prevent cancer.[126]

Garlic is the best known and most researched of the Allium vegetables and its health benefits were recognized in antiquity.[127] It has a long history of use for its possible medicinal properties, including cholesterol-lowering and cancer-preventive effects. Garlic was recently ranked the second best-selling herb in the United States.[1]

The garlic supplements available include garlic extract, aged garlic extract, allicin, and high-allicin garlic. Quercetin is also available as a supplement.

Evidence:
Cancer Survivorship
Allium compounds in garlic have potent effects against a variety of tumors.[128] Previous research showed that diallyl disulfide had potent preventive effects against cancers of the skin, colon and lung. In a recent study, diallyl disulfide caused death of leukemia cells in the laboratory, and the mechanism by which this occurred has been documented.[129] A compound derived from garlic called ajoene has also been shown to cause apoptosis, or cell death, in human leukemia cells *in vitro*.[130] Garlic extracts have been found to have direct antitumor effects when applied to prostate, bladder, colon and gastric cells.[131] In addition, garlic has also

demonstrated anti-tumor effects on transplanted cancer cells in animals.[131]

Animal studies have produced evidence that garlic can protect many body tissues from carcinogens and can inhibit cancer development, blocking cancerous changes at several stages.[132] In these studies, certain active ingredients from Allium vegetables (allyl derivatives and organosulfur compounds) inhibited cancer development in the stomach, mammary gland, esophagus, colon and lung.[126] In one study, groups of mice with bladder cancer were injected with varying concentrations of garlic or fed dilute doses of garlic in drinking water. Both subcutaneous and dietary garlic were associated with reductions in tumor number and with reduced mortality.[133]

In one 1999 study, rats with mammary tumors were fed varying doses of S-allylcysteine (SAC), a garlic component that has been associated with anti-cancer activity in previous experimental studies. In the study, SAC had no effect on tumor development or growth.[134] A different study found that shallots exhibited strong antitumor activity in mice.[135]

Allium derivatives inhibit growth of human prostate cancer cells in culture, lower secretion of PSA and enhance utilization of testosterone.[136] The water-soluble allium derivative S-allylmercaptocysteine is particularly potent against colon cancer cells in culture, when utilized together with the prostaglandin inhibitor sulindac.[137]

In an *in vitro* study with human melanoma cells, a combination of quercetin and tamoxifen were found to make tumor cells susceptible to the effects of hyperthermia (therapeutically induced fever), suggesting that such a combination may be effective against recurrent and/or metastatic melanoma.[138] Garlic has been found to inhibit tumor formation in humans by blocking the formation of powerful cancer-causing compounds called nitrosamines.[139]

A Phase I clinical trial was conducted with 14 cancer patients in which quercetin supplements seemed to show low toxicity and potential anti-tumor activity. Follow-up research will further establish if these effects are statistically significant.[140]

General Prevention Data

One study measured the effects of heating garlic on its potential anti-cancer abilities. When raw garlic was boiled or cooked in a microwave oven, the beneficial active ingredients were either partially or completely destroyed. The authors performed animal experiments and found that raw garlic reduced pre-cancerous cell abnormalities most effectively. Garlic that had been microwaved for 30 seconds was just as effective, but garlic microwaved for 60 seconds had lost all of its anti-cancer effects. However, letting the crushed raw garlic sit at room temperature for 10 minutes before microwaving preserved most of its anti-cancer effects.[132]

Two studies in China and Italy have linked garlic consumption to lower mortality from stomach cancer. Another study, the Iowa Women's Health Study, found that women who ate garlic regularly had a lower risk of colon cancer.[132] Another article reported that garlic consumption was linked to lower risk of gastric (stomach) cancer in Korea.[141]

A case-control study found that the consumption of leeks and use of garlic was associated with a reduced stomach carcinoma risk.[142] A different case-control study of 536 persons found that a high intake of Allium vegetables was associated with a reduction in risk of developing endometrial cancer.[143] A case-control study in England of 656 men found that garlic consumption significantly decreased the risk of developing prostate cancer.[144]

Quercetin, a garlic flavonoid also found in onions and apples, also appears to have anti-cancer effects. Quercetin is an antioxidant that seems to accumulate in the blood plasma if food sources are eaten frequently.[145]

Dosage and Toxicity:

The minimum quantity of garlic for reducing cancer risk is not known.[126,130] Typical doses of quercetin supplements used in trials range from 200 to 1,200 milligrams daily, and overdoses have not been reported. Quercetin supplements are contraindicated for people using cisplatin or quinolone antibiotics.[146]

CITRUS FRUITS

Citrus fruits include oranges, lemons, limes, grapefruit and tangerines. These fruits contain various phytochemicals (natural plant chemicals) that may protect against cancer. The phytochemicals being studied for possible anti-cancer effects include limonene and perillyl alcohol, which are monoterpenes, and limonoids and flavonoids. Limonene supplements are currently available.

For information on studies that have investigated the role of isolated vitamin C in cancer risk or cancer recurrence, see page 66, "Vitamin C."

For information on studies that investigated the role of modified citrus pectin (MCP), a sugar molecule found in citrus peel/pulp, see page 97, "Modified Citrus Pectin."

Evidence:
Cancer Survivorship

Limonene and perillyl alcohol have been shown to display anticarcinogenic and antitumor activity against skin, liver, lung and stomach cancers of rats *in vitro*,[147] and have been used to treat mammary and pancreatic tumors effectively in rodents.[148] This has led researchers to theorize that monoterpenes may act against human cancers at several different stages.

Another monoterpene called geraniol was found to inhibit colon cancer cell growth by 70% *in vitro*.[149] Geraniol produces these effects by interfering with certain enzymes that are critical in the formation of cancer cells. The bioflavonoids quercetin, luteolin, and kaempferol have been found to completely inhibit human prostate cancer cell growth *in vitro*.[150]

A human study known as a Phase I clinical trial was done to evaluate the effects – and determine the toxicity – of perillyl alcohol, which has shown anti-tumor effects in animals. Eighteen patients with advanced cancers took perillyl alcohol. No clear effects on the tumors were found. Stabilization of the cancer for at least 6 months was reported in some cases.[151]

Another study by the same authors used escalating doses of perillyl alcohol on continuous 4x/day basis to establish toxicity levels in 16 patients with advanced late-stage cancers. Once again, several patients showed stabilization of their cancers for more than 6 months.[152]

A Phase I study with perillyl alcohol involved 17 patients with late-stage solid tumors. A safe, non-toxic dosage was established, but this dosage did not significantly affect various measures of cancer growth.[147]

Yet another Phase I clinical trial was done to assess the toxicity and efficacy of d-limonene in 32 late-stage patients with solid tumors. Highest non-toxic doses were established and a limited Phase II trial was begun by administrating that dose to breast cancer patients. No response was observed in the Phase II trial.[153]

A case-control study in patients with a history of squamous cell carcinoma (SCC) of the skin found that the consumption of citrus peel reduced the risk of SCC recurrence.[154]

General Prevention Data

Several studies have shown that monoterpenes can prevent mammary, lung, liver and other cancers in animals.[155] Limonene in particular has been shown to prevent mammary cancer in rodents.[1]

One human study focused on limonene, which is found in citrus fruit peels. Older persons living in the southwestern United States were asked how often they ate citrus fruits, citrus juices and citrus peels. Their eating habits were compared with their rates of squamous cell skin cancer. Although skin cancer rates were not related to citrus fruit or citrus juice intakes, they were linked to citrus peel consumption. About 35% of the participants reported eating citrus peel, and they had a 34% lower risk of skin cancer than people who did not eat citrus peel. The authors concluded that citrus peel, which is rich in limonene, may protect against squamous cell skin cancer.[154]

Dosage and Toxicity:

Supplements of limonene and perillyl alcohol are not generally available. One Phase I study established a maximum tolerated dose for perillyl alcohol 4x/day as 1,200 mg/m²/dose. (At higher doses, nausea, vomiting and diarrhea occurred.) In a separate Phase I study, the maximum tolerated dose of perillyl alcohol was 1,600-2,100 mg/m² three times a day on a 14-day on/14-day off schedule. A phase I clinical study established a maximum tolerated dose for limonene as 8g/m² per day.

For dosage and toxicity information on vitamin C, see page 68.

TOMATOES AND OTHER RED OR PINK FRUITS

The red or pink color of several fruits – tomatoes, watermelon, papaya, pink guava and pink grapefruit – comes from lycopene and related compounds. Lycopene is a carotenoid. Carotenoids are natural plant chemicals that may help protect against some types of cancer.

Lycopene supplements are available and generally supply 5 to 15 milligrams of lycopene daily.

Evidence:

Cancer Survivorship

Lycopene has long been documented to exhibit potent antioxidant potential *in vitro*. This antioxidant potential is believed to be at least partially responsible for its demonstrated ability to protect cells from the kind of free radical damage that can initiate the cancer process.[156]

Recently, however, more studies have been published on lycopene's ability to inhibit later stages of the cancer process. It has been shown to inhibit proliferation of several cancer cell types, including breast, lung and endometrium.[157]

A combination of lycopene and a metabolite of vitamin D called 1-Alpha,25-dihydroxyvitamin D_3 has been found to exhibit a synergistic effect against proliferation and differentiation of leukemic cells *in vitro*.[157]

In a study involving rats with induced prostate cancer, lycopene supplementation was found to increase survival rates by 17 percent; tomato powder increased survival rates by 39%.[48]

A recent, small clinical trial involved 26 newly diagnosed prostate cancer patients. Subjects were randomly assigned to receive two 15 mg lycopene supplements/day or no supplementation for three weeks before undergoing radical prostatectomy. After surgery, the prostate glands were analyzed. In this study, lycopene supplementation seemed to be associated with a small decrease in the growth of prostate tumors.[158]

In another recent clinical study, 32 prostate cancer patients consumed tomato-sauce based pasta dishes every day (30 mg of lycopene/day) for three weeks preceding radical prostatectomy. Following the intervention, the amount of oxidative damage in the subjects blood and prostate tissue were significantly decreased. This study had no control group.[159]

General Prevention Data

Although many researchers feel that the beneficial effects of tomato products arise from several different phytochemical components, lycopene has become the focus of scientific attention for several reasons. It accounts for 50% of the carotenoids found in human blood. In *in vitro* studies, it has demonstrated an antioxidant capacity that is among the highest of the common dietary carotenoids. It has been shown to be highly tissue-specific, concentrating in the testes, adrenal gland and prostate. Many epidemiological investigations have revealed that high lycopene intake or blood levels are associated with reduced risk for cancers of the prostate, pancreas and stomach.[156]

In one study, the eating habits of over 47,000 men were recorded; the men were then followed for 6 years to see who developed prostate cancer. In the 6 years, 812 of the men were diagnosed with prostate cancer. The risk of prostate cancer was 35% lower in the men who ate the most tomato products (more than 10 servings weekly) compared with the men who ate the least (less than 1.5 servings weekly). The risk of advanced prostate cancer was reduced even more dramatically, by 53%, in the men who ate the most tomato products compared with the men who ate the least. The researchers defined tomato products as cooked tomatoes, tomato sauce, pizza and tomato juice. The study also found that diets generally high in fruits and vegetables seemed to prevent cancer.[160]

Another study looked at the influence of diet on prostate cancer risk in Greece. The researchers compared men with prostate cancer to men without cancer and found that eating tomatoes and tomato products was linked to lower prostate cancer risk. They calculated that the rate of prostate cancer in Greece could be lowered by about 40% if the population ate more tomatoes and also ate less dairy products and butter and substituted olive oil for other fats.[161]

Another study reported that higher levels of lycopene in the blood or body tissues were linked to lower risk of the following cancers: breast, cervix, skin, bladder and digestive tract. Lycopene appears to function as an antioxidant. Its antioxidant action may explain why lycopene was linked to reduced cancer risk.[1]

Dosage and Toxicity:

The average daily intake of lycopene in the U.S. is about 25 milligrams. Lycopene in processed tomato products (such as tomato sauce) is more easily absorbed than lycopene in fresh tomatoes. When lycopene supplements are taken with certain drugs (cholestyramine, colestipol, mineral oil and orlistat), absorption may be reduced.[162]

GRAPES

Grapes and grape juice are rich sources of resveratrol, a polyphenol (type of plant chemical) that may lower cancer risk. The skin of grapes contains the most resveratrol, and red and purple grapes are better sources than green grapes. Grape jam and raisins contain some resveratrol, but not as much as grapes and grape juice. Wine contains resveratrol, but alcohol has been consistently associated with increased risk for breast cancer and several other types of cancer.[1]

Resveratrol supplements are available, as are grape seed extract and grape seed powder supplements. Labels may also use the terms grape seed proanthocyanidins or procyanidins.

Evidence:
Cancer Survivorship

Purified resveratrol has been effective against human leukemia and mouse skin and mammary cancers in cell culture (not in the living body). In these experiments, resveratrol blocked cancer development at three major stages.[163]

One study tested the effects of grape seed extract on several types of human cancer cells in cell culture. The grape seed extract had toxic effects on breast, lung and stomach cancer cells, blocking their growth. Normal cells were not harmed by the grape seed extract.[164]

In several similar cellular models, resveratrol has slowed the growth of cancer cells or inhibited the formation of tumors in lymphatic, liver and breast cell lines.[165-168] Resveratrol has also triggered the death of tumors in leukemic and colon cells.[169-171]

In a recent animal study, oral administration of resveratrol was found to inhibit the growth of induced colon tumors in mice.[172] A study using human lung cancer cells found that resveratrol inhibited lung tumor growth and metastasis by interfering with the genes and their enzyme products that are responsible for the growth of these cells.[173] An *in vitro* study of human oral cancer cells found that the combination of quercetin and resveratrol led to significant inhibition of squamous cell carcinoma growth.[174]

Resveratrol has also been shown *in vitro* to make two different cervical tumor lines more susceptible to the effects of radiotherapy.[175]

General Prevention Data

Many studies have found polyphenols in general and resveratrol in particular to possess potent antioxidant and anti-inflammatory properties that are associated with preventing the kind of damage that can trigger the cancer process.[176]

Dosage and Toxicity:

No overdosage of resveratrol from dietary sources has been reported. Grape seed extract supplements usually come in doses of 50 to 100 milligrams daily. Pregnant and breast-feeding women should note that high doses of resveratrol can display estrogen-like activity in the body.[1,177,178]

DARK GREEN LEAFY AND ORANGE VEGETABLES AND FRUITS

The dark green leafy vegetables and orange fruits and vegetables are rich in carotenoids. These substances may help prevent cancer by acting as antioxidants. The carotenoids include beta-carotene, alpha-carotene, lycopene, lutein, zeaxanthin and beta-cryptoxanthin. The dark green leafy vegetables include spinach, kale, romaine lettuce, leaf lettuce, mustard greens, collard greens, chicory and Swiss chard. (These vegetables are also a rich source of alphalinolenic acid [ALA]. See the section on flax-seed on page 30 for more information about ALA and cancer.) The orange fruits and vegetables include cantaloupe, mangoes, carrots, sweet potatoes, yams, apricots, pumpkin, winter squash and bell peppers.

The available supplements include beta-carotene and extracts of vegetables such as spinach, kale, lettuce and carrots. If vegetable extracts are listed on the supplement label, the amounts of these extracts may not be shown. Beta-carotene supplements are available in various doses including 30 and 60 milligrams and 5,000 to 25,000 international units, or IUs (5,000 IUs equals 3 milligrams).

Evidence:

Cancer Survivorship

Some studies have tested whether beta-carotene supplements can help prevent cancer. One of these studies evaluated whether 50 milli grams of beta-carotene, taken daily for 5 years, would lower the rate of new skin cancers in people who had already been treated for previous skin cancers (basal cell and squamous cell types, not melanoma). In this clinical trial of 1,805 patients, beta-carotene supplements did not lower the risk of new skin cancers.[179]

A study of 79 women who had undergone surgery for breast cancer found that a high vegetable diet led to significant improvements in serum concentrations of lycopene, lutein, alpha-carotene, beta-carotene and retinol.[180] All of these factors have been identified as important elements in protection against cancer. A similar study of 224 persons with colorectal adenomas found that 20 mg of beta-carotene per day led to significant increases in serum concentrations of alpha-carotene, lycopene and beta-carotene.[181]

For more information on studies that have investigated the role of isolated carotenoids in cancer prevention and recurrence, see Chapter

Four, "Beta-Carotene," "Vitamin A" and "Vitamin C."

General Prevention Data

Many epidemiological studies have linked low blood levels of beta-carotene to high risk of cancer. In one such study, participants showed consistently low blood levels of beta-carotene for many years before they developed cancer.[182]

The international research about nutrition and cancer prevention was reviewed by a panel of leading scientists, who concluded that eating foods rich in carotenoids probably lowers the risk of lung cancer and possibly lowers the risk of cervical, breast, colorectal, stomach and esophageal cancers.[183] Another study reported that low beta-carotene intake were linked to increased lung cancer risk, and probably also increased stomach cancer risk.[184]

In the Iowa Women's Health Study, women who ate the most green leafy vegetables had less than half (44%) the risk of ovarian cancer compared with women who ate the least green leafy vegetables. The study included 29,083 postmenopausal women. Their eating habits were recorded, and then they were followed for 10 years. During this time, 139 of the women developed ovarian cancer.[185]

Dosage and Toxicity:

The average daily intake of beta-carotene in the United States is about 1.3 to 2.9 milligrams. People who consume the recommended quantities of fruits and vegetables (at least five servings daily) obtain about 3 to 6 milligrams of beta-carotene per day. Beta-carotene overdose has not been reported.[186]

Smokers should note that increased rates of lung cancer were found in smokers who took beta-carotene supplements containing 20 milligrams or more daily.[186]

VEGETABLES AND FRUITS

This chapter has included many references to research that has investigated the role of specific vegetables and fruits in preventing cancer recurrence, as well as evidence surrounding components of those foods.

The following section will detail research that has looked at overall diet, particularly overall vegetable and fruit consumption, in cancer risk and recurrence.

Diets high in vegetables and fruits have long been associated with lowered risk for cancer in general, as well as various specific types of cancer. These specific types may include cancers of the stomach, esophagus, mouth, pharynx, lung, colon, rectum, bladder, breast, prostate, pancreas and larynx.[183]

For more information on how this scientific consensus was reached, see Chapter Two.

Evidence:

Cancer Survivorship

A few clinical studies have begun to investigate how overall diets high in vegetables and fruits impact cancer patients, and many more are still in the planning stages.

In a small Phase I/Phase II clinical trial involving 11 patients with advanced lung cancer, those subjects consuming diets high in vegetables survived up to four times longer than subjects who did not follow such a diet.[187]

In a pair of small clinical studies on prostate cancer recurrence, diets high in plant foods and low in fat were combined with stress reduction techniques. In one of these studies, 10 prostate cancer patients consumed low-fat, high-fiber, plant-based diets for four months while receiving counseling on stress reduction techniques. At the end of the study, rate of PSA increase was reduced in 8 out of 10 subjects, suggesting that the combination of diet and stress reduction may be associated with slowing the rate of tumor progression in recurrent prostate cancer. This trial had no control group.[188]

In a more recent trial involving 93 prostate cancer patients that is still underway, 46 subjects were randomized to follow a low-fat, soy-supplemented, plant-based diet while engaging in stress management and exercise programs. After one year, no cancer deaths or adverse outcomes have occurred, and 80% of intervention subjects have adhered to the strict diet and lifestyle guidelines laid out in the study design.[189]

Several studies have established methods to analyze and consistently measure the various effects of overall dietary change, particularly increased vegetable and fruit consumption, among survivors of cancer.[190-192] These efforts are part of an ongoing program to evaluate the effect of diet upon survivors, and preliminary data are due soon.

General Prevention Data

There is convincing evidence that diets rich in fruits prevent cancers of the stomach, esophagus, mouth, pharynx and lung. Diets rich in vegetables prevent all of these same cancers plus colorectal cancer. Additionally, diets high in fruits *and* vegetables probably help prevent cancers of the bladder, breast, pancreas and larynx. For many other types of cancer, research completed so far suggests a protective effect of fruits and vegetables.[183]

Some studies have looked at specific groups of fruits or vegetables, such as cruciferous vegetables. Other studies have looked at total intake of fruits and vegetables. The many beneficial phytochemicals (plant chemicals) in these foods appear to protect body cells from damage that can lead to cancer or to the spread of cancer already present.[193]

In one study, 605 heart disease patients were randomized to follow either a cardioprotective Mediterranean style diet (high in vegetables, fruits and grains, low in saturated fats) or a control diet. After four years, subjects following the Mediterranean diet had a 61% lower cancer mortality rate than control subjects.[194]

Other studies have examined the effects of specific categories of phytochemicals found in vegetables and fruits. One such category, the flavonoids, have displayed a strong protective effect against stomach cancer. One case-control study done in Spain involved a total of 708 participants. The authors concluded that the well-known protective effect of fruits and vegetables against stomach cancer may be due, in part, to flavonoids.[195]

Dosage and Toxicity:

No reports of overdosage or toxicity have been documented.[187]

BEANS

Beans, also called legumes, include lentils, peas, and many types of beans (soybeans are in this category, but are discussed at the beginning of this chapter). Hummus, a spread made from chickpeas, is also in the bean category. The active ingredients in beans that may protect against cancer include saponins, protease inhibitors and phytic acid. These phytochemicals appear to protect body cells from damage that can lead to cancer. Beans are also rich in fiber, and eating plenty of fiber appears to protect against some cancers.

Evidence:

Cancer Survivorship

In cellular and animal models, saponins seem to inhibit the proliferation of cancer cells and slow the growth of tumors in various tissues. Protease inhibitors have slowed the *in vitro* and *in vivo* division of cancer cells and helped to prevent tumors from releasing substances (proteases) that destroy nearby cells. Phytic acid seems to slow the progression of cancer in lab and animal studies.[196]

A mixture of Chinese medicinal herbs called shikonin, which contains saponins, was found to reduce tumor size by more than 25% in 19 cases of late-stage lung cancer.[197] The survival time and overall quality of life was increased in these patients.

General Prevention Data

An expert panel of scientists concluded that high-fiber diets may possibly lower the risk of colorectal, pancreatic and breast cancer.[183] Another group of scientists combined the data from 13 case-control studies about diet and cancer risk. The studies included a total of over 15,000 subjects. The analysis showed that colorectal cancer risk decreased as fiber intake increased in 12 of the 13 studies. Overall, people with the highest fiber intakes had a 47% lower risk of colorectal cancer than did people with the lowest fiber intakes. The results were similar for men and women and for all age groups.[198]

Diets rich in beans, as well as fruits, vegetables and grains, reduce cancer risk according to many studies published in recent years. One case-control study included 3,237 men of various ethnic backgrounds. Men who ate the most beans had a 38% lower rate of prostate cancer than did men who ate the least beans.[36]

Dosage and Toxicity:

No overdosages have been reported for dietary sources.

WHOLE GRAINS

Whole grains are rich in fiber, vitamins and minerals, as well as hundreds of phytochemicals. The active ingredients in whole grains that may lower cancer risk include fiber (soluble and insoluble types), antioxidants, phenols, lignans, phytoestrogens (plant estrogens) and saponins. These substances, along with substances that are not yet identified, may work together to prevent diseases, including cancer.

The term "whole grain" means that all three parts of the grain kernel (germ, bran, and endosperm) are included in the food. In contrast, refined grains usually have had the bran and germ removed, leaving only the endosperm, which is high in starch. For example, white rice is refined, but brown rice is a whole grain. Other whole-grain foods include whole-wheat breads, rolls, pasta and cereals; whole-grain oat cereals such as oatmeal; popcorn; wild rice; tortillas and tortilla chips; corn; kasha (roasted buckwheat); and tabouleh (bulgar wheat).[199]

Evidence:

Cancer Survivorship

One recent study tested the effect of a wheat-bran fiber supplement on recurrence of colorectal polyps. A fiber supplement was given to men and women who had already had colorectal polyps removed. (These polyps can be precancerous.) The goal was to see if the fiber supplement prevented new polyps from forming. A total of 1,303 men and women participated. Some subjects took 2 grams daily of the fiber supplement while other subjects took 13.5 grams daily. After the subjects had taken the fiber supplements for approximately 3 years, the researchers found that the supplements had not prevented new polyps.[200]

A randomized, double-blind, placebo-controlled, Phase II study found that patients with a history of colorectal adenomas had decreased bile acid excretion rates after eating at least 13.5 grams of wheat bran per day for at least 9 months.[201] The patients also supplemented their diet with 1,500 mg of calcium per day. Researchers believe that increased concentrations and excretion rates of fecal bile acid are associated with the development of colorectal cancer.

It has been proposed that high fiber diets may decrease cancer risk in general, and specifically the growth rate of breast cancer, via several simultaneous and possibly synergistic mechanisms. Recently, researchers have proposed clinical studies to investigate the impact of supplemental fiber on growth of breast cancer, but these studies are not yet underway.[202]

General Prevention Data

There is considerable scientific evidence showing that regular consumption of whole grains lowers the risk of cancer in general and colorectal cancer in particular. A recent review of Italian case-control studies, for example, found that whole-grain consumption was linked to lower cancer risk. In these studies, the whole-grain foods most commonly consumed were whole-grain breads and whole-grain pastas.[200]

When data from 40 recent studies on whole grains and cancer risk were combined and analyzed, the risk for cancer was reduced by 34% on average in people who ate large amounts of whole grains, compared with people who ate small amounts of whole grains. Twenty different types of cancer were studied. Evidence of reduced cancer risk was found in 9 of 10 studies about colorectal cancer and polyps, 7 of 7 studies about stomach cancer, 6 of 6 studies about other digestive tract cancers, 7 of 7 studies about hormone-related cancers (such as breast and prostate cancers), 4 of 4 studies about pancreatic cancer, and 10 of 11 studies about other cancers.[203]

Dosage and Toxicity:

Very high intakes of dietary fiber or fiber supplements may lead to abdominal pain, distension and diarrhea and may possibly inhibit the absorption of some vitamins.

1 Hasler CM. Functional foods: their role in disease prevention and health promotion. Food Technology 1998; 52:57–62.

2 Presentation by Mark Messina at AICR's Nutrition after Cancer Conference, October 18, 2001, Santa Monica, CA.

3 Hendler SS, Rorvik D, eds. PDR for nutritional supplements. Montvale, NJ: Medical Economics Company Inc, 2001:428–31.

4 Barnes S, Grubbs C, Setchell KDR, et al. Soybeans inhibit mammary tumors in models of breast cancer. Mutagens and Carcinoma in the Diet, M Pariza (ed.) New York, Wiley-Liss, 1990:239-53.

5 Hawrylewicz EJ, Huang HH, Blair WH. Dietary soybean isolate and methione supplementation affect mammary tumor progression in rats. Journal of Nutrition 1991; 121:1693-8.

6 Peterson G and Barnes S. Genistein inhibition of the growth of human breast cancer cells: independence from estrogen receptors and multi-drug resistance gene. Biochem Biochemical and biophysical Resource Communications 1991; 179:661-7.

7 Barnes S and Peterson G. Biochemical targets of the isoflavone genistein in tumor cell lines. Proceedings of the Society for Experimental and Biological Medicine 1995; 208:103-8.

8 Peterson G and Barnes S. Isoflavones inhibit the growth of human prostate cancer cell lines without inhibiting epidermal growth factor receptor autophosphorylation. Prostate 1993; 22:335-45.

9 Mueller SC, Yeh Y, Chen W. Tyrosine phosphorylation of membrane proteins mediates cellular invasion of transformed cells. Journal of Cellular Biology 1992;119: 1309-25.

10 Scholar EM, Toeows ML. Inhibition of invasion of murine mammary carcinoma cells by the tyrosine kinase inhibitor genistein. Cancer Letters 1994; 87:159-62.

11 Giovanni CE, Nicoletti G, Sensi M, et al. H-2Kh and H-2Dh gene transfections in B16 melanoma differently affect nonimmuno-logical properties relevant to the metastatic process. International Journal of Cancer 1994; 59:269-74.

12 Messina MJ, et al. Soy intake and cancer risk: a review of the in vitro and in vivo data. Nutrition and Cancer 1994; 21:113-31.

13 Hawrylewicz EJ, Zapata JJ, Blair WH. Soy and experimental cancer: animal studies. Journal of Nutrition 1995; 125:698S–708S.

14 Su S, Lai M, Yeh T, et al. Overexpression of HER-2/neu enhances the sensitivity of human bladder cancer cells to urinary isoflavones. European Journal of Cancer 2001; 37:1413–8.

15 Su SJ, Yeh TM, Lei HY, et al. The potential of soybean foods as a chemoprevention approach for human urinary tract cancer. Clinical Cancer Research 2000; 6(1):230-6.

16 Wang SY, Yang KW, Hsu YT, Chang CL, Yang YC. The differential inhibitory effects of genistein on the growth of cervical cancer cells in vitro. Neoplasma 2001; 48:227-33.

17 Lin Y, Yee JA, McGuire MH, et al. Effect of dietary supplementation of soybeans on experimental metastasis of melanoma cells in mice. Nutrition and Cancer 1997; 29(1):1-6.

18 Menon LG, Kuttan R, Nair MG, et al. Effect of isoflavones genistein and daidzein in the inhibition of lung metastasis in mice induced by B16F-10 melanoma cells. Nutrition and Cancer 1998; 30(1):74-7.

19 Nagata C. Ecological study of the association between soy product intake and mortality from cancer and heart disease in Japan. International Journal of Epidemiology 2000; 29:832–6.

20 Kennedy AR, Wan XS. Effects of the Bowman-Birk inhibitor on growth, invasion, and clonogenic survival of human prostate epithelial cells and prostate cancer cells. Prostate 2002; 50(2):125-33.

21 Stoll BA. Eating to beat breast cancer: potential role for soy supplements. Annals of Oncology 1997; 8:223-5.

22 Evans BA, Griffiths K, Morton MS. Inhibition of 5 alpha-reductase in genital skin fibroblasts and prostate tissue by dietary lignans and isoflavonoids. Journal of Endocrinology 1995; 147:295-302.

23 Moyad MA. Soy, disease prevention, and prostate cancer. Seminars in Urologic Oncology 1999; 17:97–102.

24 Hillman GG, Forman JD, Kucuk O, et al. Genistein potentiates the radiation effect on prostate carcinoma cells. Clinical Cancer Research 2001; 7:382–90.

25 Messina MJ, Loprinzi CL. Soy for breast cancer survivors: a critical review of the literature. Journal of Nutrition 2001; 131:3095S–108S.

26 Khoshyomn S, Manske GC, Lew SM, et al. Synergistic action of genistein and cisplatin on growth inhibition and cytotoxicity of human medulloblastoma cells. Pediatric Neurosurgery (Switzerland) 2000; 33(3):123-31.

27 Wan XS, Hamilton TC, Ware JH, et al. Growth inhibition and cytotoxicity induced by Bowman-Birk inhibitor concentrate in cisplatin-resistant human ovarian cancer cells. Nutrition and Cancer 1998; 31(1): 8-17.

28 Zhang L, Wan XS, Donahue JJ, et al. Effects of the Bowman-Birk inhibitor on clonogenic survival and cisplatin- or radiation-induced cytotoxicity in human breast, cervical and head and neck cancer cells. Nutrition and Cancer 1999; 33(2):165-73.

29 Santell RC, Kieu N, Helfereich WG. Genistein inhibits growth of estrogen-independent human breast cancer cells in culture but not in athymic mice. Journal of Nutrition 2000; 130(7):665-9.

30 Sun AS, et al. Pilot study of a specific dietary supplement in tumor-bearing mice and in stage IIIB and IV non-small cell lung cancer. Nutrition and Cancer 2001; 39:85-95.

31 Hsieh CY, Santell RC, Haslam SZ et al. Estrogenic effects of genistein on the growth of estrogen receptor positive human breast cancer (MCF-7) cells in vitro and in vivo. Cancer Research 1998; 58:3833-8.

32 McMichael-Phillips DF, Harding C, Morton M, et al. Effects of soy-protein supplementation on epithelial proliferation in the histologically normal human breast. American Journal of Clinical Nutrition 1998; 68(suppl):1431S -5S.

33 Petrakis NL, Barnes S, King EB, et al. Stimulatory influence of soy protein isolate on breast fluid secretion in pre- and postmenopausal women. Cancer Epidemiology Biomarkers and Prevention 1996; 5:785-94.

34 Pollard M, Wolter W. Prevention of spontaneous prostate-related cancer in Lobund-Wistar rats by a soy protein isolate/isoflavone diet. Prostate 2000; 45:101-5.

35 Jacobsen BK, Knutsen SF, Fraser GE. Does high soy milk intake reduce prostate cancer incidence? The Adventist Health Study (United States). Cancer Causes and Control 1998; 9:553-7.

36 Kolonel LN, Hankin JH, Whittemore AS, et al. Vegetables, fruits, legumes and prostate cancer: a multiethnic case-control study. Cancer Epidemiology, Biomarkers and Prevention 2000; 9:795-804.

37 Nagata C, Takatsuka N, Shimizu H, et al. Effect of soymilk consumption on serum estrogen and androgen concentrations in Japanese men. Cancer Epidemiology, Biomarkers and Prevention 2001; 10:179-84.

38 Habito RC, Montalto J, Leslie E, et al. Effects of replacing meat with soyabean in the diet on sex hormone concentrations in healthy adult males. British Journal of Nutrition 2000; 84:557-63.

39 Urban D, Irwin W, Kirk M, et al. The effect of isolated soy protein on plasma biomarkers in elderly men with elevated serum prostate specific antigen. Journal of Urology 2001; 165:294-300.

40 Kishida T, Beppu M, Nashiki K, et al. Effect of dietary soy isoflavone aglycones on the urinary 16alpha-to-2-hydroxyestrone ratio in C3H/HeJ mice. Nutrition and Cancer 2000; 38:209-14.

41 Lu L-J W, Anderson KE, Grady JJ, et al. Decreased ovarian hormones during a soya diet: implications for breast cancer prevention. Cancer Research 2000; 60:4112-21.

42 This P, De la Rochefordiere A, Clough K, et al. Phytoestrogens after breast cancer. Endocrine-Related Cancer 2001; 8:129-34.

43 Lamartiniere CA. Protection against breast cancer with genistein: a component of soy. American Journal of Clinical Nutrition 2000; 71:1705S-7S.

44 Shu XO, Jin F, Dai Q. Soyfood intake during adolescence and subsequent risk of breast cancer among Chinese women. Cancer Epidemiology, Biomarkers and Prevention 2001; 10:483 8.

45 Dai Q, Shu XO, Jin F, et al. Population-based case-control study of soyfood intake and breast cancer risk in Shanghai. British Journal of Cancer 2001; 85:372-8.

46 De la Taille A, Katz A, Vacherot F, et al. Cancer of the prostate: influence of nutritional factors. A new nutritional approach. Presse Med 2001; 30(11):561-4.

47 Anderson WF, Hawk E, Berg CD. Secondary chemoprevention of upper aerodigestive tract tumors. Seminars in Oncology 2001; 28(1):106-20.

48 Boileau TW, Clinton SK, Liao Z, et al. Lycopene, tomato powder and dietary restriction influence survival of rats with prostate cancer induced by NMU and testosterone. Journal of Nutrition 2001; 131:191S-99S.

[49] Clarke RG, Lund EK, Latham P, et al. Effect of eicosapentaenoic acid on the proliferation and incidence of apoptosis in the colorectal cell line HT29. Lipids 1999; 34(12):1287-95.

[50] Hubbard NE, Lim D, Erickson KL. Alteration of murine mammary tumorigenesis by dietary enrichment with n-3 fatty acids in fish oil. Cancer Letters 1998; 124(1):1-7.

[51] Rose DP, Connolly JM. Effects of dietary omega-3 fatty acids on human breast cancer growth and metastasis in nude mice. Journal of the National Cancer Institute 1993; 85(21):1743-7.

[52] Rose DP, Connolly JM. Dietary fat and breast cancer metastasis by human tumor xenografts. Breast Cancer Research and Treatment 1997; 46(2-3):225-37.

[53] Pandalai PK, Pilat MJ, Yamazaki K, et al. The effects of omega-3 and omega-6 fatty acids on in vitro prostate cancer growth. Anticancer Research 1996; 16(2):815-20.

[54] Good CK, Lasko CM, Adam J, et al. Diverse effect of fish oil on the growth of aberrant crypt foci and tumor multiplicity in F344 rats. Nutrition and Cancer 1998; 31(3):204-11.

[55] Mukutmoni-Norris M, Hubbard NE, Erickson KL. Modulation of murine tumor vasculature by dietary n-3 fatty acids in fish oil. Cancer Letters 2000; 150(1):101-9.

[56] Ravichandran D, Cooper A, Johnson CD. Effect of 1-(gamma)linolenyl-3-eicosapentaenoyl propane diol on the growth of human pancreatic carcinoma in vitro and in vivo. European Journal of Cancer 2000; 36:423-7.

[57] Hardman WE, Avula CP, Fernandes G, et al. Three percent dietary fish oil concentrate increased efficacy of doxorubicin against MDA-MB 231 breast cancer xenografts. Clinical Cancer Research 2001; 7:2041-9.

[58] Yam D, Peled A, Shinitzky M. Suppression of tumor growth and metastasis by dietary fish oil combined with vitamins E and C and cisplatin. Cancer Chemotherapy and Pharmacology 2001; 47:34-40.

[59] Ogilvie GK, Fettman MJ, Mallinckrodt CH, et al. Effect of fish oil, arginine, and doxorubicin chemotherapy on remission and survival time for dogs with lymphoma: a double-blind, randomized placebo-controlled study. Cancer 2000; 88(8):1916-28.

[60] Rose DP, Connolly JM, Coleman M. Effect of omega-3 fatty acids on the progression of metastases after the surgical excision of human breast cancer cell solid tumors growing in nude mice. Clinical Cancer Research 1996; 2(10):1751-6.

[61] Griffini P, Fehres O, Klieverik L, et al. Dietary omega-3 polyunsaturated fatty acids promote colon carcinoma metastasis in rat liver. Cancer Research 1998; 58:3312-19.

[62] Salem ML, Kishihara K, Abe K, et al. N-3 polyunsaturated fatty acids accentuate B16 melanoma growth and metastasis through suppression of tumoricidal function of T cells and macrophages. Anticancer Research (Greece) 2002; 20(5A)3195-203.

[63] Bradley MO, et al. Tumor targeting by covalent conjugation of a natural fatty acid to paclitaxel. Clinical Cancer Research 2001; 7:3229-38.

[64] Bougnoux P, et al. Cytotoxic drugs efficacy correlates with adipose tissue docosahexaenoic acid level in locally advanced breast carcinoma. British Journal of Cancer 1999; 79:1765-9.

[65] Presentation by Dr. Lilian Thompson at AICR's Nutrition after Cancer Conference, October 18, 2001, Santa Monica, CA.

[66] Gogos CA, Ginopoulos P, Zoumbos NC, et al. The effect of dietary omega-3 polyunsaturated fatty acids on T-lymphocyte subsets of patients with solid tumors. Cancer Detection and Prevention 1995; 19(5):415-17.

[67] Gogos CA, Ginopoulos P, Salsa B, et al. Dietary omega-3 polyunsaturated fatty acids plus vitamin E restore immunodeficiency and prolong survival for severely ill patients with generalized malignancy: a randomized control trial. Cancer 1998; 82(2):395-402.

[68] Barber MD, Ross JA, Preston T, et al. Fish oil-enriched nutritional supplement attenuates progression of the acute-phase response in weight-losing patients with advanced pancreatic cancer. Journal of Nutrition 1999; 129(6):1120-5.

[69] Gogos CA, Skoutelis A, Kalfarentzos F. The effects of lipids on the immune response of patients with cancer. Journal of Nutrition Health and Aging 2000; 4(3):172-5.

[70] Wigmore SJ, Barber MD, Ross JA, et al. Effect of oral eicosapentaenoic acid on weight loss in patients with pancreatic cancer. Nutrition and Cancer 2000; 36(2):177-84.

71 Barber MD. Cancer cachexia and its treatment with fish-oil-enriched nutritional supplementation. Nutrition 2001; 17(9):751-5.

72 Gramaglia A, Loi GF, Mongioj V, et al. Increased survival in brain metastatic patients treated with stereotactic radiotherapy, omega three fatty acids and bioflavonoids. Anticancer Research 1999; 19(6C):5583-6.

73 Terry P, Lichtenstein P, Feychting M, et al. Fatty fish consumption and risk of prostate cancer. Lancet 2001; 357:1764-6.

74 Petrik MB, McEntee MF, Johnson BT, et al. Highly unsaturated (n-3) fatty acids, but not alpha-linolenic, conjugated linoleic or gamma-linolenic acids, reduce tumorigenesis in Apc(Min/+) mice. Journal of Nutrition 2000; 130:2434-43.

75 Bartsch H, Nair J, Owen RW. Dietary polyunsaturated fatty acids and cancers of the breast and colorectum: emerging evidence for their role as risk modifiers. Carcinogenesis 1999; 20:2209-18.

76 Hendler SS, Rorvik D, eds. PDR for nutritional supplements. Montvale, NJ: Medical Economics Company Inc, 2001: 145-50.

77 Burns CP, Halabi S, Clamon GH, et al. Phase I clinical study of fish oil fatty acid capsules for patients with cancer cachexia: cancer and leukemia group B study 9473. Clinical Cancer Research 1999; 5(12):3942-7.

78 Thompson LU, Robb P, Serraino M, et al. Mammalian lignan production from various foods. Nutrition and Cancer 1991; 16:43-52.

79 Haggans CJ, Hutchins AM, Olson BA, et al. Effect of flaxseed consumption on urinary estrogen metabolites in postmenopausal women. Nutrition and Cancer 1999; 33:188-95.

80 Tou JC, Thompson LU. Exposure to flaxseed or its lignan component during different developmental stages influences rat mammary gland structures. Carcinogenesis 1999; 20:1831-5.

81 Rickard SE, Yuan YV, Thompson LU. Plasma insulin-like growth factor I levels in rats are reduced by dietary supplementation of flaxseed or its lignan secoisolariciresinol diglycoside. Cancer Letters 2000; 161:47-55.

82 Phipps WR, Martini MC, Lampe JW, et al. Effect of flax seed ingestion on the menstrual cycle. Journal of Clinical Endocrinology and Metabolism 1993; 77:1215-9.

83 Haggans CJ, Travelli EJ, Thomas W, et al. The effect of flaxseed and wheat bran consumption on urinary estrogen metabolites in premenopausal women. Cancer Epidemiology, Biomarkers and Prevention 2000; 9:719-25.

84 Demark Wahnefried W, Price DT, Polascik TJ, et al. Pilot study of dietary fat restriction and flaxseed supplementation in men with prostate cancer before surgery: exploring the effects on hormonal levels, prostate-specific antigen, and histopathologic features. Urology 2001; 58:47-52.

85 Lewis NM, Seburg S, Flanagan NL. Enriched eggs as a source of n-3 polyunsaturated fatty acids for humans. Poultry Science 2000; 79:971-4.

86 Tou JC, Chen J, Thompson LU. Flaxseed and its lignan precursor, secoisolariciresinol diglycoside, affect pregnancy outcome and reproductive development in rats. Journal of Nutrition 1998; 128:1861-8.

87 Hendler SS, Rorvik D, eds. PDR for nutritional supplements. Montvale, NJ: Medical Economics Company Inc, 2001: 150-2.

88 Thompson LU. Experimental studies on lignans and cancer. Bailliere's Clinical Endocrinology and Metabolism 1998; 12(4):691-705.

89 Jenab M, Thompson LU. The influence of flaxseed and lignans on colon carcinogenesis and beta-glucuronidase activity. Carcinogenesis 1996; 17(6):1343-8.

90 Rickard SE, Yuan YV, Thompson LU. Plasma insulin-like growth factor I levels in rats are reduced by dietary supplementation of flaxseed or its lignans secoisolariciresinol diglycoside. Cancer Letters 2000; 161(1):47-55.

91 Jenab M, Rickard SE, Orcheson LJ. Flaxseed and lignans increase cecal beta-glucuronidase activity in rats. Nutrition and Cancer 1999; 33(2):154-8.

92 Takasaki M, Konshima T, Komatsu K, et al. Anti-tumor-promoting activity of lignans from the aerial part of Saussurea medusa. Cancer Letters 2000; 158(1):53-9.

93 Yan L, Yee JA, Li D, et al. Dietary flaxseed supplementation and experimental metastasis of melanoma cells in mice. Cancer Letters 1998; 124(2):181-6.

94 Menendez JA, et al. Effects of gamma-linolenic acid and oleic acid on paclitaxel cytotoxicity in human breast cancer cells. European Journal of Cancer 2001; 37:402-13.

95 Thompson LU, Rickard SE, Orcheson LJ, et al. Flaxseed and its lignan and oil components reduce mammary tumor growth at a late stage of carcinogenesis. Carcinogenesis 1996; 17(6):1373-6.

96 Rickard SE, Yuan YV, Chen J, et al. Dose effects of flaxseed and its lignan on N-methyl-N-nitrosourea-induced mammary tumorigenesis in rats. Nutrition and Cancer 1999; 35(1):50-7.

97 Thompson LU, Rickard SE, Cheung F, et al. Variability in anticancer lignan levels in flaxseed. Nutrition and Cancer 1997; 27(1): 26-30.

98 Simon HB, ed. Good for the heart but not for the prostate? The alpha-linolenic acid dilemma. Harvard Men's Health Watch 2002; 6(6):1-3.

99 Dufresnse CJ, Farnworth ER. A review of latest research findings on the health promotion properties of tea. The Journal of Nutritional Biochemistry 2001; 12:404-21.

100 Ahmad N, Mukhtar H. Green tea polyphenols and cancer: biologic mechanisms and practical implications. Nutrition Reviews 1999; 57:78-83.

101 Pianetti S, Guo S, Kavangh KT, et al. Green tea polyphenol epigallocatechin-3-gallate inhibits Her-2/neu signaling, proliferation, and transformed phenotype of breast cancer cells. Cancer Research 2002; 62(3):652-5.

102 Otsuka T, Ogo T, Eto T, et al. Growth inhibition of leukemic cells by (-)-epigallocatechin gallate, the main constituent of green tea. Life Sciences 1998; 63(16):1397-1403.

103 Liu J, Chen SH, Lin CL, et al. Inhibition of melanoma growth and metastasis by combination with (-)-epigallocatechin-3-gallate and dacarbazine in mice. Journal of Cellular Biochemistry 2001; 83(4):631-42.

104 Uesato S, et al. Inhibition of green tea catechins against the growth of cancerous human colon and hepatic epithelial cells. Cancer Letters 2001; 170:41-4.

105 Guangjin N, Chaofang J, Yuanlin C, et al. Distinct effects of tea catechins on 6-hydroxydopamine-induced apoptosis in PC12 cells. Archives of Biochemistry and Biophysics 2002; 397(1):84-90.

106 Li HC, Yashiki S, Sonada J, et al. Green tea polyphenols induce apoptosis in vitro in peripheral blood T lymphocytes of adult T-cell leukemia patients. Japanese Journal of Cancer Research 2000; 91(1):34-40.

107 Zhou JR, Yu L, Zhong Y, et al. Soy and tea as functional foods in prevention of prostate cancer progression. American Journal of Clinical Nutrition 2002; 75(2S):408S-409S.

108 Hirose M, et al. Prevention by antioxidants of heterocyclic amine-induced carcinogenesis in a rat medium-term liver bioassay: results of extended and combination treatment experiments. European Journal of Cancer Prevention 1998; 7:61-7.

109 Liao S, et al. Growth inhibition and regression of human prostate and breast tumors in athymic mice by tea epigallocatechin gallate. Cancer Letters 1995; 96:239-43.

110 August DA, et al. Ingestion of green tea rapidly decreases prostaglandin E2 levels in rectal mucosa in humans. Cancer Epidemiology, Biomarkers and Prevention 1999; 8:709-13.

111 Nakachi K, Suemasu K, Suga K, et al. Influence of drinking green tea on breast cancer malignancy among Japanese patients. Japanese Journal of Cancer Research 1998; 89(3):254-261.

112 Inoue M, Tajima K, Mizutani M, et al. Regular consumption of green tea and the risk of breast cancer recurrence: follow up study from the Hospital-based Epidemiologic Research Program at Aichi Cancer Center, Japan. Cancer Letters 2001; 167(2):175-82.

113 Berger SJ, Gupta S, Belfi CA, et al. Green tea constituent (-)-epigallocatechin-3-gallate inhibits topoisomerase I activity in human colon carcinoma cells. Biochemical and Biophysical Research Communications 2001; 288(1):101-5.

114 Shukla Y, Taneja P. Anticarcinogenic effect of black tea on pulmonary tumors in Swiss albino mice. Cancer Letters 2002; 176(2):137-41.

115 Dreosti IE, Wargovich MJ, Yang CS. Inhibition of carcinogenesis by tea: the evidence from experimental studies. Critical Reviews in Food Science and Nutrition 1997; 37:761-70.

116 Yang CS, Wang ZY. Tea and cancer. Journal of the National Cancer Institute 1993; 85:1038-49.

117 Hendler SS, Rorvik D, eds. PDR for nutritional supplements. Montvale, NJ: Medical Economics Company Inc, 2001: 202-6.

118 Finley JW, Ip C, Lisk DJ, et al. Cancer-protective properties of high-selenium broccoli. Journal of Agricultural Food Chemistry 2001; 49(5):2679-83.

119 Srivastava B, Shukla Y. Antitumor promoting activity of indole-3-carbinol in mouse skin carcinogenesis. Cancer Letters 1998; 134(1):91-5.

120 Brignall MS. Prevention and treatment of cancer with indole-3-carbinol. Alternative Medicine Review 2001; 6:580-9.

121 Clapper ML, Szarka CE, Pfieffer GR, et al. Preclinical and clinical evaluation of broccoli supplements as inducers of glutathione S-transferase activity. Clinical Cancer Research 1997; 3(1):25-30.

122 Rosen CA, Woodson GE, Thompson JW, et al. Preliminary results of the use of indole-3-carbinol for recurrent respiratory papillomatosis. Otolaryngology and Head and Neck Surgery 1998; 118(6):810-15.

123 Bell MC, et al. Placebo-controlled trial of indole-3-carbinol in the treatment of CIN. Gynecologic Oncology 2000; 78:123-9.

124 Verhoeven DT, Goldbohm RA, van Poppel G, et al. Epidemiological studies on brassica vegetables and cancer risk. Cancer Epidemiology, Biomarkers and Prevention 1996; 5:733-48.

125 Michaud DS, Spiegelman D, Clinton SK, et al. Fruit and vegetable intake and incidence of bladder cancer in a male prospective cohort. Journal of the National Cancer Institute 1999; 91:605-13.

126 Bianchini F, Vainio H. Allium vegetables and organosulfur compounds: do they help prevent cancer? Environmental Health Perspectives 2001; 109:893-902.

127 Rivlin RS. Historical perspective on the use of garlic. Journal of Nutrition 2001; 131:951S-4S

128 Pinto JT, Rivlin RS. Garlic and other allicin vegetables in cancer prevention. In: Heber D, Blackburn GL and Go VLM, eds. Nutritional Oncology (San Diego, Academic Press): 393-403, 1999.

129 Kwon KB, Yoo SJ, Ryu DG, et al. Induction of apoptosis by diallyl disulfide through activation of capsase-3 in human leukemia HL-60 cells. Biochemistry and Pharmacology 2002; 63:41-7.

130 Ahmed N, et al. Ajoene, a garlic-derived natural compound, enhances chemotherapy-induced apoptosis in human myeloid leukemia CD34-positive resistant cells. Anticancer Research 2001; 21:3519-23.

131 Lamm DL, Riggs DR. Enhanced immunocompetence by garlic: role in bladder cancer and other malignancies. Journal of Nutrition 2001; 131:1067S-70S.

132 Song K, Milner JA. The influence of heating on the anticancer properties of garlic. Journal of Nutrition 2001; 1054S-7S.

133 Riggs DR, DeHaven JI, Lamm DL. Allium sativum (garlic) treatment for murine transitional cell carcinoma. Cancer 1997; 79(10):1987-94.

134 Cohen LA, Zhao Z, Pittman B, et al. S-allylcysteine, a garlic constituent, fails to inhibit N-methylnitrosourea-induced rat mammary tumorigenesis. Nutrition and Cancer 1999; 35(1):58-63.

135 Caldes G, Prescott B. A potential antileukemic substance present in Allium ascalonicum. Planta Medica 1973; 23:99-100.

136 Pinto JT, Qiao CH, Xing J, et al. Alterations of prostate biomarker expression and testosterone utilization in human LNCaP prostatic carcinoma cells by garlic-derived S-allylmercaptocysteine. Prostate 2001; 45:304-14.

137 Shirin H, Pinto JT, Kawabata Y, et al. Antiproliferative effects of S-allylmercaptocysteine on colon cancer cells, when tested alone or in combination with sulindac sulfide. Cancer Research 2002; In press.

138 Piantelli M, Tatone D, Castrilli G, et al. Quercetin and tamoxifen sensitize human melanoma cells to hyperthermia. Melanoma Research 2001; 11(5):469-76.

139 Mei X. The blocking effect of garlic on the formation of N-nitrosoprolinc in the human body. Acta Nutrilogica Sinica 1989; 11:144-5.

140 Ferry DR, Smith A, Malkhandi J, et al. Phase I clinical trial of the flavonoid quercetin: pharmacokinetics and evidence for in vivo tyrosine kinase inhibition. Clinical Cancer Research 1996; 2:659-68.

141 Kim HJ, Chang WK, Kim MK, et al. Dietary factors and gastric cancer in Korea: a case-control study. International Journal of Cancer 2002; 97:531-5.

142 Dorant E, et al. Consumption of onions and a reduced risk of stomach carcinoma. Gastroenterology 1996; 110:12-20.

143 Xiao Ou Shu, et al. A population-based case-control study of dietary factors and endometrial cancer in Shanghai, People's Republic of China. American Journal of Epidemiology 1993; 137:155-65.

144 Key TJA, et al. A case-control study of diet and prostate cancer. British Journal of Cancer 1997; 76:678-87.

145 Hollman PC, van Trijp JM, Mengelers MJ, et al. Bioavailability of the dietary antioxidant flavonol quercetin in man. Cancer Letters 1997; 114:139–40.

146 Hendler SS, Rorvik D, eds. PDR for nutritional supplements. Montvale, NJ: Medical Economics Company Inc, 2001: 390–3.

147 Hudes GR, Szarka CE, Adams A, et al. Phase I pharmacokinetic trial of perillyl alcohol (NSC 641066) in patients with refractory solid malignancies. Clinical Cancer Research 2000; 6(8):3071-80.

148 Crowell PL. Monoterpenes in breast cancer chemoprevention. Breast Cancer Research and Treatment 1997; 46:191–7.

149 Carnesecchi S, et al. Geraniol, a component of plant essential oils, inhibits growth and polyamine biosynthesis in human colon cancer cells. Journal of Pharmacology and Experimental Therapeutics 2001; 298:197-200.

150 Knowles LM, et al. Flavonoids suppress androgen-independent human prostate tumor proliferation. Nutrition and Cancer 2000; 38:116-22.

151 Ripple GH, Gould MN, Stewart JA, et al. Phase I clinical trial of perillyl alcohol administered daily. Clinical Cancer Research 1998; 4:1159–64.

152 Ripple GH, Gould MN, Arzoomanian RZ, et al. Phase I clinical and pharmacokinetic study of perillyl alcohol administered four times a day. Clinical Cancer Research 2000; 6(2):390-6.

153 Vigushin DM, Poon GK, Boddy A. Phase I and pharmacokinetic study of D-limonene in patients with advanced cancer. Cancer Chemotherapy and Pharmacology 1998; 42(2):111-7.

154 Hakim IA, Harris RB, Ritenbaugh C. Citrus peel use is associated with reduced risk of squamous cell carcinoma of the skin. Nutrition and Cancer 2000; 37:161-8.

155 Gould MN. Cancer chemoprevention and therapy by monoterpenes. Environmental Health Perspectives 1997; 105:977–9.

156 Gerster H. The potential role of lycopene for human health. Journal of American College of Nutrition 1997; 16(2):109-26.

157 Amir H, Karas M, Giat J, et al. Lycopene and 1,25-dihydroxyvitamin D3 cooperate in the inhibition of cell cycle progression and induction of differentiation in HL-60 leukemic cells. Nutrition and Cancer 1999; 33(1):105-12.

158 Kucuk O, Sarkar FH, Sakr W, et al. Phase II randomized clinical trial of lycopene supplementaition before radical prostatectomy. Cancer Epidemiology Biomarkers and Prevention 2001; 10(8):861-8.

159 Chen L, Stacewicz-Sapuntzakis M, Duncan C, et al. Oxidative DNA damage in prostate cancer patients consuming tomato sauce-based entrees as a whole-food intervention. Journal of the National Cancer Institute 2001; 93(24):1872-9.

160 Giovannucci E, Ascherio A, Rimm EB, et al. Intake of carotenoids and retinol in relation to risk of prostate cancer. Journal of the National Cancer Institute 1995; 87:1767–76.

161 Bosetti C, Tzonou A, Lagiou P, et al. Fraction of prostate cancer incidence attributed to diet in Athens, Greece. European Journal of Cancer Prevention 2000; 9:119–23.

162 Hendler SS, Rorvik D, eds. PDR for nutritional supplements. Montvale, NJ: Medical Economics Company Inc, 2001: 284–7.

163 Jang M, Cai L, Udeani GO, et al. Cancer chemopreventive activity of resveratrol, a natural product derived from grapes. Science 1997; 275:218–20.

164 Ye X, Krohn RL, Liu W, et al. The cytotoxic effects of a novel IH636 grape seed proanthocyanidin extract on cultured human cancer cells. Molecular and Cellular Biochemistry 1999; 196:99–108.

165 Koide T, Kamei H, Hashimoto Y, et al. Antitumor effect of hydrolyzed anthocyanin from grape rinds and red rice. Cancer Biotherapy and Radiopharmaceuticals 1996; 11(4):273-7.

166 Delmas D, Jannin B, Malki MC, et al. Inhibitory effect of resveratrol on the proliferation of human and rat hepatic derived cell lines. Oncology Reports 2000; 7(4)847-52.

167 Agarwal C, Sharma Y, Zhao J, et al. A polyphenolic fraction from grape seeds causes irreversible growth inhibition of breast carcinoma MDA-MB468 cells by inhibiting mitogen-activated protein kinases activation and inducing G1 arrest and differentiation. Clinical Cancer Research 2000; 6(7)2921-30.

168 De Ledinghen V, Monvoisin A, Neaud V. Trans-resveratrol, a grapevine-derived polyphenol, blocks hepatocyte growth factor-induced invasion of hepatocellular carcinoma cells. International Journal of Oncology 2001; 19(1):83-8.

169 Clement MV, Hirpara JL, Chawdhury SH, et al. Chemopreventive agent resveratrol, a natural product derived from grapes, triggers CD95 signaling-dependent apoptosis in human tumor cells. Blood 1998; 93(3):996-1002.

170 Surh YJ, Hurh YJ, Kang JY, et al. Resveratrol, an antioxidant present in red wine, induces apoptosis in human promyelocytic leukemia (HL-60) cells. Cancer Letters 1999; 140(1-2):1-10.

171 Mahyar-Roemer M, Katsen A, Mestres P, et al. Resveratrol induces colon tumor cell apoptosis independently of p53 and preceded by epithelial differentiation, mitochondrial proliferation and membrane potential collapse. International Journal of Cancer 2001; 94(5):615-22.

172 Schneider Y, Duranton B, Gosse F, et al. Resveratrol inhibits intestinal tumorigenesis and modulates host-defense-related gene expression in an animal model of human familial adenomatous polyposis. Nutrition and Cancer 2001; 39(1):102-7.

173 Mollerup S, Ovrebo S, Haugen A. Lung carcinogenesis: resveratrol modulates the expression of genes involved in the metabolism of PAH in human bronchial epithelial cells. International Journal of Cancer 2001; 92:18-25.

174 el Attar TM, Virji AS. Modulating effect of resveratrol and quercetin on oral cancer growth and proliferation. Anticancer Drugs 1999; 10:187-93.

175 Zoberi I, Bradbury CM, Curry HA, et al. Radiosensitizing and anti-proliferative effects of resveratrol in two human cervical tumor cell lines. Cancer Letters 2002; 175(2):165-73.

176 Jang M, Cai L, Udeani GO, et al. Cancer chemopreventive activity of resveratrol, a natural product derived from grapes. Science 1997; 275:218-20.

177 Hendler SS, Rorvik D, eds. PDR for nutritional supplements. Montvale, NJ: Medical Economics Company Inc, 2001: 397-401.

178 Hendler SS, Rorvik D, eds. PDR for nutritional supplements. Montvale, NJ: Medical Economics Company Inc, 2001: 200-2.

179 Greenberg ER, Baron JA, Stukel TA, et al. A clinical trial of beta-carotene to prevent basal-cell and squamous-cell cancers of the skin. The Skin Cancer Prevention Study Group. New England Journal of Medicine 1990; 323:789-95.

180 Rock CL, et al. Responsiveness of carotenoids to a high vegetable diet intervention designed to prevent breast cancer recurrence. Cancer Epidemiology Biomarkers Prevention 1997; 6:617-23.

181 Wahlqvist ML, et al. Changes in serum carotenoids in subjects with colorectal adenomas after 24 months of beta-carotene supplementation. Australian Polyp Prevention Project Investigators. American Journal of Clinical Nutrition 1994 Dec; 60:936-43.

182 Wald N. Retinol, beta-carotene and cancer. Cancer Surveys 1987; 6:635-51.

183 World Cancer Research Fund and American Institute for Cancer Research. Food, nutrition, and the prevention of cancer: a global perspective. American Institute for Cancer Research, 1997: 506.

184 van Poppel G, Goldbohm RA. Epidemiologic evidence for beta-carotene and cancer prevention. American Journal of Clinical Nutrition 1995; 62:1393S-402S.

185 Kushi LH, Mink PJ, Folsom AR, et al. Prospective study of diet and ovarian cancer. American Journal of Epidemiology 1999; 149:21-31.

186 Hendler SS, Rorvik D, eds. PDR for nutritional supplements. Montvale, NJ: Medical Economics Company Inc, 2001: 36-42.

187 Sun AS, Ostadal O, Ryznar V, et al. Phase I/II study of stage II and IV non-small cell lung cancer patients taking a specific dietary supplement. Nutrition and Cancer 1999; 34(1):62-9.

[188] Saxe GA, Hebert JR, Carmody JF, et al. Can diet in conjunction with stress reduction affect the rate of increase in prostate specific antigen after biochemical recurrence of prostate cancer? Journal of Urology 2001; 166(6):2202-7.

[189] Ornish D, Lee KL, Fair WR, et al. Dietary trial in prostate cancer: Early experience and implications for clinical trial design. Urology 2001; 57(4S1):200-1.

[190] Rock CL, Moskowitz A, Hulzar B, et al. High vegetable and fruit diet intervention in premenopausal women with cervical intraepithelial neoplasia. Journal of the American Dietetic Association 2001; 101(10):1167-74.

[191] Pierce JP, Faerber S, Wright FA, et al. Feasibility of a randomized trial of a high-vegetable diet to prevent breast cancer recurrence. Nutrition and Cancer 1997; 28(3):282-8.

[192] Rock C. Antioxidants in dietary intervention to prevent cervical cancer and breast cancer recurrence. Free Radical Biology and Medicine 2000; 29(S1):S7.

[193] Abdulla M, Gruber P. Role of diet modification in cancer prevention. Biofactors 2000; 12:45-51.

[194] De Lorgeril M, Salen P, Martin JL, et al. Mediterranean dietary pattern in a randomized trial prolonged survival and possible reduced cancer risk. Archives of Internal Medicine 1998; 158(1):1181-7.

[195] Garcia-Closas R, Gonzalez CA, Agudo A, et al. Intake of specific carotenoids and flavonoids and the risk of gastric cancer in Spain. Cancer Causes and Control 1999; 10:71-5.

[196] Gould MN. Prevention and therapy of cancer by monoterpenes. Journal of Cellular Biochemistry 1995; S22:139-44.

[197] Guo XP, Zhang XY, Zhang SD. Clinical trial on the effects of shikonin mixture on later stage lung cancer. Zhong Xi Yi Jie He Za Zhi 1991; 11:598-9.

[198] Howe GR, Benito E, Castelleto R, et al. Dietary intake of fiber and decreased risk of cancers of the colon and rectum: evidence from the combined analysis of 13 case-control studies. Journal of the National Cancer Institute 1992; 84:1887-96.

[199] Slavin JL, Jacobs D, Marquart L, et al. The role of whole grains in disease prevention. Journal of the American Dietetic Association 2001; 101:780-5.

[200] Alberts DS, Martinez ME, Roe DJ, et al. Lack of effect of a high-fiber cereal supplement on the recurrence of colorectal adenomas. The New England Journal of Medicine 2000; 342:1156-62.

[201] Alberts DS, et al. Randomized, double-blinded, placebo-controlled study of the effect of wheat bran fiber and calcium on fecal bile acids in patients with resected adenomatous colon polyps. Journal of the National Cancer Institute 1996; 17:81-92.

[202] Stoll BA. Can supplementary dietary fibre suppress breast cancer growth? British Journal of Cancer 1996; 73(5):557-9.

[203] Jacobs DR Jr, Marquart L, Slavin J, et al. Whole-grain intake and cancer: an expanded review and meta-analysis. Nutrition and Cancer 1998; 30:85-96.

Chapter Four

Vitamins and Minerals

Although a great deal is known about the nutritional requirements of humans, there is still much that is not known with certainty. Research in this area is a continual process, and the Recommended Daily Allowances (RDAs) will continue to evolve as our knowledge of nutrient requirements expand. Moreover, because RDAs are designed to provide an estimate of the amount of a nutrient needed to prevent nutrient deficiency (and deficiency-related diseases), they only provide part of the picture – they do not, for example, attempt to define the optimum intake level of a nutrient.

Recently, the National Academy of Sciences has established Tolerable Upper Intake Levels (ULs) for several nutrients, which represent the maximum total daily dosage that is "likely to pose no risk of adverse effects." Where applicable, these amounts can be found under "Dosage and Toxicity" below.

Although it might appear that ensuring a healthful dose of vitamins and minerals has become more complicated, the basic guidelines still hold true: eat a diet containing a wide variety of plant-based foods. Supplements of vitamins and other essential nutrients are not a substitute for a healthy diet, but they are important for survivors who cannot obtain optimal intakes through diet alone.

Because so little science exists on the period of time during which tumor tissue undergoes active chemotherapy or radiation treatment, it is advisable to avoid high doses of antioxidants during this period until more is known.

Note: Several of the studies listed below involve very large doses of nutrients, but these levels were administered in tightly controlled and closely monitored clinical settings. For those not undergoing treatment, the benefits of antioxidant

*vitamins and minerals at high levels are under study and the scientific infor-
mation in this chapter can help you and your doctor decide on the best course of
action for you.*

VITAMIN A

The term vitamin A refers to a number of related compounds called
retinoids, including retinol, retinal and retinoic acid. It is involved with
important functions in the body including vision, reproduction, cell growth
and immunity.

Evidence:
Cancer Survivorship

In laboratory studies, retinoids have been shown to inhibit the growth
of some types of cancer. In *in vitro* studies, researchers have found that
retinoic acid inhibits the growth of some but not all types of oral and
breast cancer cells.[1,2] In animal studies, some retinoids have been shown
to inhibit various types of cancer, but they can produce toxic effects.[3] A
study of human gastric cells inoculated into mice found that the administration of all-trans retinoic acid, a form of vitamin A, led to significant
inhibition of tumor formation and the metastasis of the transplanted
cells.[4]

Animal studies in rats have found that several derivatives of vitamin
A, such as 13-*cis* retinoic acid, 9-*cis* retinoic acid and Ro 13-6307, have
anti-tumor effects inside the animal.[5]

A patient with acute myeloid leukemia was induced to complete
remission by using 60 mg per day of oral all-trans retinoic acid.[6] A study
of 11 patients with chronic myeloid leukemia found that all-trans retinoic
acid combined with standard interferon therapy was superior to interferon therapy alone.[7] A study of 5 patients with acute promyelocytic
leukemia found that the administration of 45 mg all-trans retinoic acid
twice per day for 21 days led to remission in all patients after a median
of 3 months.[8] A study of 72 patients with acute promyelocytic leukemia
found that all-trans retinoic acid is an effective therapy for this type of
leukemia and can be considered a first-choice treatment in some cases.[9]

A retrospective study of 44 children with acute promyelocytic leukemia who were treated with all-trans retinoic acid or conventional therapy
found that those who had received all-trans retinoic acid followed by
chemotherapy had significantly better disease status than those who

received conventional therapy alone.[10] In addition, the overall survival rate and event-free survival rate were significantly better than the conventional treatment group.

In people with a history of squamous cell or basal cell skin cancer or actinic keratoses (a risk factor for skin cancer), daily supplementation with 25,000 IU of retinol for up to 5 years reduced the development of new squamous cell cancers, but not basal cell cancers.[11]

In a study involving 2,592 patients with head and neck cancer or lung cancer, most of whom were previous or current smokers, the researchers found that very large doses of vitamin A for 2 years (150,000 to 300,000 IU of retinyl palmitate daily) did not affect survival rates.[12] Retinyl palmitate in daily doses of 200,000 IU for 1 year was also found to have no significant effect on the rate of recurrence of head and neck cancers.[13]

In several studies, vitamin A has been shown to inhibit precancerous lesions in the mouth. In one of these studies, weekly supplements of 200,000 IU of vitamin A for 6 months increased remission of existing precancerous lesions in the mouth and inhibited the formation of new lesions in people who chewed tobacco or betel nuts.[14]

In one study, daily supplements of 30,000 IU of vitamin A, plus 1 gram of vitamin C and 70 milligrams of vitamin E reduced the recurrence rate of adenomas in the large bowel, a risk factor for colon cancer.[15]

Small clinical studies for patients at risk for superficial bladder cancer have been undertaken, but no results have yet been published.

General Prevention Data

Intake of vitamin A from food and supplements has not been shown to affect the risk of ovarian cancer or bladder cancer. Results have varied from studies investigating whether there is an association between retinol intake or blood retinol levels and breast or lung cancer risk.[11-13]

The Beta-Carotene and Retinol Efficacy Trial studied over 18,000 people who were smokers, former smokers or workers exposed to asbestos.[16] About half of the people were given daily supplements of 30 milligrams of beta-carotene and 25,000 IU of retinol. After about 4 years of supplementation, the study was stopped earlier than planned when it was discovered that the supplemented group had a 28% higher rate of lung cancer than the non-supplemented group.

Dosage and Toxicity:

For adults, the current dietary recommendations for vitamin A are:

Men, age 19 and older: 900 micrograms (3,000 IU)

Women, age 19 and older: 700 micrograms (2,330 IU)

Pregnant women, age 19 and older: 770 micrograms (2,565 IU)

Breastfeeding women, age 19 and older: 1,300 micrograms (4,335 IU)

Doses used in supplementation studies investigating cancer risk have typically been between 25,000 IU to 300,000 IU per day, much higher than recommended amounts. The UL for Vitamin A is 3,000 micrograms, meaning that intake higher than 3,000 micrograms (10,000 IU) per day can be toxic, resulting in liver abnormalities, bone loss and other adverse effects. Pregnant women and women who may become pregnant should note that high doses of vitamin A can cause birth defects.

VITAMIN D

Vitamin D has many functions in the body including the regulation of calcium levels in the blood. In addition to being a dietary component, it is synthesized by the skin through sun exposure, and many authorities believe that this is as important a source of Vitamin D as diet.

Evidence:

Cancer Survivorship

In laboratory studies, vitamin D has been shown to inhibit the growth of some types of cancer. In an *in vitro* study, researchers found that vitamin D inhibited the growth of 2 types of breast cancer cells.[17] Vitamin D has also been shown to reduce prostate cancer cell growth in *in vitro* studies. A form of vitamin D_3 analog has been found to induce apoptosis, or cell death, in several colorectal carcinoma cell lines.[18] This analog, when combined with another form of vitamin D, has been found to arrest the growth of thyroid carcinoma cells.[19] An additional study found that this form of vitamin D_3 completely inhibited the growth of human head and neck squamous cell carcinoma lines transplanted in mice.[20]

In a small human study, calcitriol (a form of vitamin D) slowed the progression of prostate cancer in 7 men as measured by prostate specific antigen (PSA) levels.[21] A study of 11 men with advanced prostate cancer found that weekly administration of calcitriol combined with the standard chemotherapeutic agent docetaxel led to PSA reductions of more than 50% in 5 patients.[22]

In another small study, 6 out of 7 men with prostate cancer responded favorably to treatment with calcitriol.[23] However, in a similar study, only 2 out of 13 men responded favorably.[24] In each of these studies, doses of calcitriol were high enough to cause undesirable side effects.

A metabolite of vitamin D in the body called 1-alpha, 25-dihydroxyvitamin D_3 has been found to slow the rise of PSA levels in selected patients with early recurrent prostate cancer.[25] This vitamin D metabolite has also been found to decrease the ability of prostate cancer cells to adhere to other cells and to prevent the migration of cancer cells to other parts of the body.[26] 1-alpha, 25-dihydroxyvitamin D_3 has also been shown to inhibit the growth of Kaposi's sarcoma, a neoplasm often associated with AIDS infections, in laboratory studies.[27] This metabolite, given in doses of 1 to 1.5 micrograms per day and combined with cis-retinoic acid, led to clinical responses in 61% of patients with a bone marrow dysplasia disorder.[28]

A Phase I clinical trial involving patients with head and neck carcinoma found that 1-alpha, 25-dihydroxyvitamin D_3 reduced the presence of CD34 cells, which are known to reduce the ability of the body to fight cancer cell growth.[29] The researchers found that the use of this vitamin D metabolite improved the overall immune system function of patients with head and neck carcinoma. A different study found that this metabolite increased the survival rate of patients with osteosarcoma compared to a control group, but this difference was not statistically significant.[30]

Another chemical analog of vitamin D called alfacalcidol was studied in a group of 11 patients with brain tumors.[31] This Phase II clinical trial found that 0.04 micrograms per kilogram of body weight of this vitamin D analog given daily to these brain tumor patients led to significant regression in 20% of malignant glioma cases. Alfacalcidol was administered along with a standard surgery-radiation-chemotherapy regimen.

General Prevention Data

Several studies have shown that breast cancer risk decreases in areas closer to the equator. It is believed that this may be due to increased sunlight exposure, especially in the winter, resulting in increased vitamin D synthesis. In northern regions, winter sunlight is ineffective in stimulating skin synthesis of Vitamin D. Consumption of diets rich in vitamin D as well as higher blood levels of vitamin D have also been associated with lower breast cancer risk in white women.[32,33]

Higher blood levels of vitamin D have been associated with decreased risk of colorectal adenomas, a risk factor for colon cancer. Although not all studies have agreed, a review of several studies suggested that an intake of about 160 IU of vitamin D per day or more has been associated with about a 32% reduction in colon cancer risk.[34]

Increased sun exposure as well as higher blood levels of vitamin D have been associated with reduced prostate cancer risk. Several studies have investigated a possible connection between the consumption of dairy products including milk and increased prostate cancer risk, though this association remains controversial. If an association exists, it may be related to reduced vitamin D levels in the body since increased calcium intake reduces the body's production of vitamin D.[35]

Dosage and Toxicity:
For adults, the current dietary recommendations for vitamin D are:
Age 19-50: 5 micrograms (200 IU)
Age 51-69: 10 micrograms (400 IU)
Age 70 and older: 15 micrograms (600 IU)
Vitamin D can be toxic at high doses. The UL for Vitamin D is 50 micrograms, meaning that intake higher than 50 micrograms (2,000 IU) per day can cause a number of health problems including raising blood levels of calcium, which can result in heart rhythm abnormalities and other serious complications.

VITAMIN C

Vitamin C, also called ascorbic acid, has a number of important roles in the body. It functions primarily as an antioxidant, protecting cells from the damaging effects of free radicals. The damage caused by free radicals may lead to the development of many types of cancer. Under certain conditions, however, vitamin C may also serve as a prooxidant.

Evidence:
Cancer Survivorship
Studies conducted years ago by Linus Pauling and colleagues proposed that very large doses of vitamin C, given in shots and taken orally, increase the survival time of people with terminal cancer.[36] However, results from two other studies showed that supplementation with 10 grams of vitamin C per day did not affect disease progression or survival

time of people with advanced colorectal cancer or other advanced cancers.[37,38]

In laboratory studies, vitamin C has been shown to be toxic to many types of cancer cells. However, there is evidence that the concentrations of vitamin C that are toxic to cancer cells can only be achieved by intravenous (given with a shot) administration of vitamin C.[39] Other research suggests that vitamin C inhibits gastric cancer cell growth at concentrations similar to those in gastric juice.[40] *In vitro* studies have shown that the form of vitamin C used by the body enters cancer cells via glucose transporters on the cell membrane, where it accumulates and – at least theoretically – may actually stimulate cancer growth.[41]

Vitamin C combined with vitamin B_{12} has been found to be toxic to human larynx carcinoma cells.[42] This toxic effect occurred when both vitamins were administered separately at levels that are nontoxic to normal cells.

The results from one study showed that daily supplements of 1 gram of vitamin C, plus 30,000 IU of vitamin A and 70 milligrams of vitamin E reduced the recurrence rate of adenomas in the large bowel. A randomized, double-blind study of 36 patients with large bowel adenomas who received 3 grams of vitamin C per day found that those who received vitamin C had a significant reduction in the number of polyps compared to the placebo group.[43] A study of 24 patients with oral leukoplakia and 24 patients with primary oral cancer who had undergone radical resection of the lesion found that a combination of vitamin C, vitamin E, and beta-carotene led to a general improvement in several parameters in 97.5% of the study population.[44]

A randomized double-blind clinical trial of 137 patients with colorectal polyps, recognized precursors of colorectal cancer, found that supplementation with vitamins C and E led to a small reduction in the rate of polyp recurrence following surgical removal.[45]

In another population of people with precancerous stomach lesions, daily supplementation with 2 grams of vitamin C for 6 years increased regression of the lesions.[46] A retrospective study of 1,826 patients who had reached an incurable stage of cancer found that those who had received vitamin C at some stage of their illness had a median overall survival time that was nearly twice as long as those who had never received vitamin C supplementation.[47] A study in Japan among 99 terminal cancer patients found similar results with the exception that the vitamin C group had a median survival time that was nearly six times as long as those who did not receive supplementation.[48]

General Prevention Data

Many studies have reported a link between diets rich in vitamin C and lower cancer risk, including cancers of the lung, stomach, colon-rectum, oral cavity, larynx-pharynx and esophagus. Higher blood levels of vitamin C have also been associated with reduced risk of many forms of cancer. In general, a protective effect of vitamin C appears to occur with intakes of 80 to 110 milligrams per day or more.[49]

In people without a history of colorectal adenomas, daily supplementation with 1 gram of vitamin C plus 400 milligrams of vitamin E for 4 years did not affect the incidence of adenomas.[50] In a large study involving over 700,000 people, the use of vitamin C supplements did not affect the risk of death from colorectal cancer.[51]

Laboratory studies show that vitamin C inhibits the formation of carcinogenic compounds in the stomach.[52] One study examined the effects of daily supplementation with 120 milligrams of vitamin C and 30 micrograms of molybdenum in a large population of Chinese people at high risk for stomach and esophageal cancer.[53] The researchers found that the supplements did not affect the risk of stomach or esophageal cancer.

Dosage and Toxicity:

For adults, the current dietary recommendations for vitamin C are:
Men, age 19 and older: 90 milligrams
Men who smoke: 125 milligrams
Women, age 19 and older: 75 milligrams
Women who smoke: 110 milligrams
Pregnant women, age 19 and older: 85 milligrams
Breastfeeding women, age 19 and older: 120 milligrams

Dietary intake recommendations for vitamin C are higher for smokers than non-smokers because smoking is known to cause cell damage and deplete vitamin C from the body. The UL for adult consumption of Vitamin C is 2,000 milligrams/day.

Doses used in supplementation studies have varied greatly, from 120 milligrams to 10 grams (10,000 milligrams) of vitamin C per day. In general, smaller doses have been used in studies investigating whether vitamin C is protective against cancer while higher doses have been used for cancer treatment.

The most common side effect from high doses of vitamin C (more than 2,000 milligrams per day) is diarrhea. For more information about antioxidant use during treatment, see page 2.

BETA-CAROTENE

Beta-carotene is a carotenoid that can be converted by the body into vitamin A. It acts as an antioxidant, protecting cells from the damaging effects of excess free radicals. The damage caused by free radicals may lead to the development of many types of cancer. Beta-carotene may also improve immune function.

Evidence:
Cancer Survivorship:
In *in vitro* studies, researchers have found that beta-carotene inhibits the growth of some but not all types of breast cancer cells.[1] At least one study has found that high concentrations of beta-carotene induces apoptosis, or cell death, in colon adenocarcinoma cell lines.[54] At this writing, however, only a few studies have investigated how beta-carotene affects the promotion and progression of tumors in animal subjects. One such study involving mouse subjects transplanted with human mammary cancer showed that beta-carotene inhibited tumor growth and prolonged survival.[55]

In a study involving people who had previously had cancer of the oral cavity, pharynx or larynx, supplementation with 50 milligrams of beta-carotene per day for about 4 years did not significantly affect the recurrence of these cancers, nor did it significantly affect the rate of the development of lung cancer.[56]

In another study, researchers examined the effects of daily supplements of 50 milligrams of beta-carotene for 5 years in people who had had a recent non-melanoma skin cancer.[57] The beta-carotene supplements did not affect the rates of new non-melanoma skin cancers.

Several studies have shown that beta-carotene alone or in combination with other antioxidants may inhibit precancerous lesions in the mouth and stomach. One of these studies examined the effects of daily supplementation with 30 milligrams of beta-carotene for 6 years in people with precancerous stomach lesions. The researchers found that the beta-carotene supplements increased regression of the precancerous lesions.

A multicenter, double-blind, placebo-controlled trial of 50 patients with oral leukoplakia, a premalignant lesion, found that 60 mg/day of beta-carotene produced a significant clinical response in 52% of the treated group.[58] In addition, those receiving beta-carotene had an improvement of at least one grade of dysplasia in 39% of cases.

General Prevention Data

A number of studies have found associations between diets rich in beta-carotene and lower rates of many forms of cancer, especially lung cancer.[59]

One study examined the effects of daily supplementation with 15 milligrams of beta-carotene in combination with 50 micrograms of selenium and 30 milligrams of alpha-tocopherol (vitamin E) in a large population of Chinese people at high risk for stomach and esophageal cancer. The researchers found that the supplements reduced the rate of death from stomach cancer. In another study involving over 39,000 females, women receiving 50 milligrams of beta-carotene supplements every other day for approximately 2 years did not have lower rates of any forms of cancer than those receiving a placebo.[60] Similarly, another large study found that 50 milligrams of beta-carotene supplements taken every other day for 12 years did not affect the rates of any forms of cancer in men.[61] In a population of people in Australia, daily supplementation with 30 milligrams of beta-carotene for 4½ years did not affect the risk of basal cell or squamous cell skin cancer.[62] Daily supplements of 25 milligrams of beta-carotene have also been shown to have no affect on the prevention of colorectal adenomas in healthy people.

The Beta-Carotene and Retinol Efficacy Trial studied over 18,000 people who were smokers, former smokers or workers exposed to asbestos. About half of the people were given daily supplements of 30 milligrams of beta-carotene and 25,000 IU of retinol (vitamin A). After about 4 years of supplementation, the study was stopped earlier than planned when it was discovered that the supplemented group had a 28% higher rate of lung cancer than the non-supplemented group. Another study reported similar results in over 29,000 male smokers. Men given daily supplements of 20 milligrams of beta-carotene for 5 to 8 years experienced an 18% higher rate of lung cancer.[63] These men also experienced a 23% higher rate of prostate cancer than those not receiving supplements.[64]

Dosage and Toxicity:

There are no recommended dietary intake or upper intake levels for beta-carotene. Unlike vitamin A, which is toxic at high doses, excess beta-carotene does not cause the same symtoms of toxicity. Doses used in supplementation studies investigating cancer risk have typically been between 20 and 50 milligrams of beta-carotene, taken daily or every other day.

For more information about antioxidants during cancer treatment, see page 2.

SELENIUM

Selenium is a mineral that acts as an antioxidant, protecting cells from the damaging effects of free radicals. The damage caused by free-radicals may lead to the development of many types of cancer. Selenium is also involved with proper immune function and has other effects on cancer prevention.

Evidence:

Cancer Survivorship

In several laboratory studies, selenium has been shown to inhibit the growth of some types of cancer. An *in vitro* study showed that selenomethionine (a form of selenium) inhibited the growth of three types of breast, prostate and skin cancer cells.[65] In rats, selenium was shown to inhibit both the formation and growth of transplanted human breast tumors.[66] A different study in rats found that selenium has an important affect on the inhibition of certain enzymes that are critical in the development of cancer.[67]

A study of 32 patients with brain tumors that had previously been treated with surgery, chemotherapy or radiation found that 1,000 micrograms of selenium administered daily in saline solution led to a definite improvement in the general condition of the patients.[68] All of the patients had improvement in erythrocyte, thrombocyte and hemoglobin measures.

A study of 32 women age 32 to 81 years old with breast cancer found that a supplementation protocol of vitamin C, vitamin E, beta-carotene and 387 micrograms of selenium daily reduced the risk of metastasis, improved quality of life, led to partial remission in 6 patients and reduced the risk of cancer mortality in the group.[69] A study of patients with precancerous and malignant oral lesions found that serum selenium levels were significantly lower in the malignant group than in the precancerous group and a control group.[70] The precancerous group then received three 4-week cycles of selenium. Out of 18 patients in this group, 2 had complete responses, 5 had partial responses, 6 had minor responses and five had stable disease after the therapy was completed.

A randomized, controlled clinical trial of 1,312 patients with a history of skin cancer were given daily oral supplementation of 200 micrograms/day of selenium or placebo.[71] The patients were assessed at 6 to 12 month intervals for several years. The researchers found significant reductions in total cancer mortality and reduced incidence of prostate, colorectal, lung and total cancers in the treatment group.

General Prevention Data

Studies have shown higher rates of some forms of cancer in geographic areas with low soil selenium levels, a factor affecting the selenium content of food grown in those areas. In addition, there have been a number of studies linking higher selenium levels in the body with reduced rates of several forms of cancer including prostate, colorectal, lung, esophageal and gastric cardia cancer.[59] One of these studies involving over 33,000 men found an association between higher levels of selenium in the men's toenails (an indication of selenium intake) with lower risk of advanced prostate cancer.[72] In a study that analyzed selenium levels in the blood, researchers found that low selenium levels were associated with a 4- to-5-fold increased risk of prostate cancer.[73] Another study found an association between higher levels of toenail selenium and lower risk of colon cancer, but no association between levels of toenail selenium and the risk of breast or prostate cancer.[74]

In a large study involving over 62,000 females, no association was found between selenium levels in the women's toenails and cancer risk, including cancers of the breast, uterus, colon, skin, ovary or lung.[75,76]

One study examined the effects of daily supplementation with 50 micrograms of selenium in combination with 30 milligrams of alpha-tocopherol (vitamin E) and 15 milligrams of beta-carotene in a large population of Chinese people at high risk for stomach and esophageal cancer.[53] The researchers found that the supplements reduced the rate of death from stomach cancer. An examination of the same population of people found that higher blood levels of selenium were associated with lower risk of esophageal and gastric cardia cancer.

In men with hepatitis B infection, a known risk factor for liver cancer, daily supplementation with 200 micrograms of selenium for 4 years reduced the risk of liver cancer.[77] Another study involving Chinese men living in a high risk area for liver cancer found that daily supplementation with a higher dose (500 micrograms) of selenium for 3 years also reduced the risk of liver cancer.[78]

The National Cancer Institute has initiated a large prostate cancer prevention trial involving over 32,000 men.[79] This study, which was launched in 2001 and will take about 12 years to complete, will examine the effects of daily supplementation with 200 micrograms of selenium and 400 milligrams (400 IU) of vitamin E on prostate cancer risk.

Dosage and Toxicity:

For adults, the current dietary recommendations for selenium are:
Age 19 and older: 55 micrograms
Pregnant women: 60 micrograms
Breastfeeding women: 70 micrograms

Doses used in most supplementation studies investigating cancer risk have been 200 micrograms of selenium per day. There is a narrow margin of safety with selenium supplements. Selenium is toxic at high doses (more than 400 micrograms per day) and can cause hair loss, nausea, diarrhea, brittle nails and nervous system problems.

For more information about antioxidant use during treatment, see page 2.

VITAMIN E

Vitamin E exists in 8 different forms – 4 tocopherols and 4 tocotrienols. The most active form is alpha-tocopherol, or α-tocopherol, which acts as an antioxidant, protecting cells from the damaging effects of free radicals. The damage caused by free radicals may lead to the development of many types of cancer. Vitamin E may also improve immune function and block the formation of some carcinogens in the body.

Evidence:

Cancer Survivorship

Vitamin E has been shown to inhibit cancer growth in animal and in *in vitro* studies,[80] though responses vary depending on the form of vitamin E and the type of cancer cell. Tocotrienols have been shown to inhibit growth of some types of human breast cancer cells.[81] In addition, vitamin E succinate, a derivative of vitamin E, and alpha-tocopherol have been shown to promote apoptosis (cell death) in some types of human prostate cancer cells.[82,83] An alternative form of vitamin E called alpha-tocopheryl acetate has been shown to have apoptotic and anti-tumor forming effects on malignant cells.[84]

Vitamin E may offer modest protection against the recurrence of colorectal adenomas. One study found that daily supplements of 70 milligrams of vitamin E, plus 30,000 IU of vitamin A and 1 gram of vitamin C reduced the recurrence rate of adenomas in the large bowel.[15] In people without a history of colorectal adenomas, daily supplementation with 400 milligrams of vitamin E plus 1 gram of vitamin C for 4 years did not affect the incidence of adenomas.[50]

A randomized, controlled trial found that patients with generalized malignancy who received a formulation combining vitamin E and omega-3 polyunsaturated fatty acids had improved immune system function and prolonged survival compared to a placebo group.[85] These patients were severely ill and were considered malnourished as a result of the malignancy prior to the intervention.

General Prevention Data

Some studies have found an association between diets rich in vitamin E and slightly reduced risk of breast cancer. A recent review of 118 studies on vitamin E and breast cancer concluded that supplemental vitamin E has not been shown to offer protection against breast cancer.[86] Higher blood levels of vitamin E have been associated with lower lung cancer risk in some studies, but one large study found no association between vitamin E intake and lung cancer risk in men.[87]

There is conflicting evidence on whether vitamin E intake is associated with lower colon cancer risk, though there may be some benefit in women.[88,89]

One study examined the effects of daily supplementation with 30 milligrams of alpha-tocopherol in combination with 15 milligrams of beta-carotene and 50 micrograms of selenium in a large population of Chinese people at high risk for stomach and esophageal cancer.[53] The researchers found that the supplements reduced the rate of death from stomach cancer. Results from another study involving over 1 million people showed that regular use of vitamin E supplements did not affect the risk of death from stomach cancer.[51]

Two large studies have shown that supplemental vitamin E reduces the risk of fatal prostate cancer in male smokers. In one of these studies involving over 29,000 male smokers, men supplemented with 50 milligrams (50 IU) of vitamin E daily for 5 to 8 years experienced a slightly lower rate of colorectal cancer and a 32% lower rate of prostate cancer than those not receiving supplements.[90,64] In addition, deaths due to prostate cancer were 41% lower in the supplemented group. However, the vitamin E supplements slightly increased the risk of pancreatic, stomach and bladder cancer (although these increases were not statistically significant).

In 2001, the National Cancer Institute initiated a large prostate cancer prevention trial involving over 32,000 men.[79] This study will take about 12 years to complete and will examine the effects of daily supplementation with 400 milligrams (400 IU) of vitamin E and 200 micrograms of selenium on prostate cancer risk.

A few studies have investigated whether vitamin E offers protection against the development of other cancers including oral, pharyngeal, esophageal, bladder, cervical, ovarian and pancreatic cancer. However, results from these studies have been inconsistent.[91-102]

Dosage and Toxicity:

For adults, the current dietary recommendations for vitamin E are:

Age 19 and older (including pregnant women): 15 milligrams (22 IU)
Breastfeeding women: 19 milligrams (28 IU)

These values are based on the α-tocopherol form of vitamin E because it is the most prevalent form in the body. The α-tocopherol form is found in vitamin E supplements made completely from natural sources (frequently labeled as RRR-α-tocopherol or d-α-tocopherol). Some forms of synthetic vitamin E supplements are not quite as active (frequently labeled as all-rac-α-tocopherol or dl-α-tocopherol). For these forms, 1 milligram of vitamin E equals only about 1 IU.

Doses used in supplementation studies investigating cancer risk have typically ranged from 50 IU to 400 IU of vitamin E per day.

In general, vitamin E has a low risk of toxicity. However, vitamin E in very high doses thins the blood, which can result in excessive bleeding, hemorrhage or stroke. For adults, it has been recommended to limit consumption to less than 1,000 milligrams (1,500 IU) of vitamin E (α-tocopherol) per day. However, little is known about health problems resulting from long-term use of doses close to this value.

It should be noted that a deficiency of zinc in the diet has been shown to reduce the amount of vitamin E in the blood.[103]

For more information about antioxidant use during therapy, see page 2.

CALCIUM

Calcium is the most abundant mineral in the body and is the main structural component of bones and teeth.

Evidence:
Cancer Survivorship

In two calcium supplementation studies, people with a history of colorectal adenomas received supplements of 1,200 milligrams or 2,000 milligrams of calcium per day for several years.[104,105] The calcium supplements had a modest protective effect against recurrence of the adenomas. Conversely, in a similar study, supplementation for 6 months with 2,000 milligrams of calcium per day, in addition to vitamins, did not have a protective effect on another measure of colorectal cancer risk.[106]

General Prevention Data

Animal and *in vitro* studies suggest that calcium may inhibit the development of colorectal cancer.[107] Several studies in humans have found associations between increased calcium intake and slightly reduced risk of colorectal cancer.

Some studies have suggested a possible link between consumption of dairy products and increased risk of prostate cancer, suggesting that either fat or calcium is the culprit. However, this association remains controversial. A recent study examining the dietary habits of over 20,000 men reported that increased dairy product and calcium intakes were associated with increased risk of prostate cancer.[108] Conversely, another large study found no association between total calcium intake or consumption of dairy products and prostate cancer risk.[109] If an association exists, it may be related to reduced vitamin D levels in the body since increased calcium intake reduces the body's production of 1,25-dihydroxyvitamin D, the most active form of the vitamin.[35]

Dosage and Toxicity:

For adults, the current dietary recommendations for elemental calcium are:

Age 19-50: 1,000 milligrams

Age 51 and older: 1,200 milligrams

Doses used in supplementation studies investigating colorectal cancer risk have typically been between 1,200 and 2,000 milligrams of calcium per day.

Excess calcium intake (generally more than 2,500 milligrams of calcium per day) can cause kidney stones, constipation and intestinal gas.

FOLIC ACID

Folic acid and folate are two forms of a B vitamin that is involved in the formation of new cells and the prevention of neural tube defects, a type of birth defect. Folic acid is the form contained in supplements and fortified foods. Folate is the form that is naturally present in food. Because of its involvement with the synthesis and repair of DNA and other actions, a folate deficiency could cause DNA damage and lead to cancer.

Evidence:

Cancer Survivorship

A placebo-controlled, randomized study of 20 patients with colonic adenomas found that those patients who received 5 mg/day of folate had accelerated improvement after 6 months compared to the placebo group. This improvement was determined in part by measuring folate concentrations in serum, red blood cells and in the mucosa of the colon. The researchers also found that another key indicator of disease progression was significantly improved after 6 months.[110]

Several controlled clinical studies have shown that supplementation with 10 mg/day of folic acid can normalize smears taken from patients with a history of cervical dysplasia. The regression rates from cervical dysplasia in these studies ranged from 20% to 100%.[111-116]

General Prevention Data

Results from several studies suggest that dietary folate intake from food or supplements is associated with lower risk of colorectal adenomas and colorectal cancer.[117] One large study showed that women who took multivitamins containing folic acid for at least 15 years were 75% less likely to develop colon cancer than those who did not.[118] There is also evidence that folic acid supplements may offer some protection against colon cancer in people with ulcerative colitis and in those who consume more than two alcoholic drinks per day.

Two large studies have suggested an association between increased dietary folate intake and reduced breast cancer risk in women who consume alcoholic beverages. This has been studied because alcohol consumption is believed to increase breast cancer risk. In one of these studies, scientists investigated the dietary habits of over 88,000 women. For women who consumed one or more alcoholic beverages per day, folic acid intake of at least 600 micrograms per day from food and supplements reduced breast cancer risk by about half compared with women who consumed less than 300 micrograms of folic acid per day.[119] For women who consumed less than one alcoholic beverage per day, there was no association between folic acid intake and reduction of breast cancer risk. Another study conducted in China involving women who did not regularly consume alcohol found that high folate intake from food was associated with lower breast cancer risk.[120]

In men, results from two studies suggest that folate intake from food and supplements may reduce the risk of lung cancer, especially in smokers. Based on several human studies, it is uncertain whether folate intake from food or supplements affects the risk of cervical cancer.[117]

Dosage and Toxicity:

For adults, the current dietary recommendations for folic acid are:
Age 19 and older: 400 micrograms
Pregnant women: 600 micrograms
Breastfeeding women: 500 micrograms

Folic acid has a low risk of toxicity, but high folic acid intakes can mask a vitamin B_{12} deficiency. For adults, it is recommended to limit consumption of folic acid from supplements and fortified foods to less than 1,000 micrograms (1 milligram) per day.

Folic acid supplements may interfere with certain drugs, such as methotrexate, that are used to treat cancer.

IRON

Iron is a mineral that has a variety of important functions in the body including the formation of healthy red blood cells and muscle cells and proper immune function.

However, it is believed that excess iron may increase the formation of free radicals, causing oxidative damage to tissue in the colon and other tissues.

Evidence:

General Prevention Data

A number of *in vitro, in vivo* and human studies have suggested that iron intake from food or supplements as well as body stores of iron are associated with increased risk of colorectal cancer.[121]

Of 11 studies in humans examining a possible association between iron and colorectal cancer, 9 showed that iron intake was associated with increased risk of colorectal cancer.

One of these studies involving over 14,000 people found that increased dietary consumption of iron was associated with increased colon cancer risk in both men and women.[122] Consumption of red meat, an excellent source of iron, has also been linked to increased colorectal cancer risk, but it is not clear whether the iron content or something else, such as fat, is the culprit.

Dosage and Toxicity:

For adults, the current dietary recommendations for iron are:

Men, age 19 and older: 8 milligrams

Premenopausal Women: 18 milligrams

Postmenopausal Women: 8 milligrams

Pregnant women, age 19-50: 27 milligrams

Breastfeeding women, age 19-50: 9 milligrams

Iron can be toxic at high doses. It is important to keep iron-containing dietary supplements out of children's reach since iron overload can be fatal to children. For adults, it is recommended to limit consumption of iron to only the recommended doses.

THIAMIN

Thiamin, or thiamine, is a B vitamin that is required for the proper function of many important enzymes in the body. A thiamin deficiency causes a variety of serious problems since it affects the cardiovascular, muscular, nervous and gastrointestinal systems.

Evidence:
Cancer Survivorship
Studies indicate that the growth of cancer tumors may deplete the body of thiamin. Thus, cancer patients are frequently supplemented with thiamin to prevent thiamin deficiency.[123]

However, one study involving mice found that thiamin supplementation at doses of 25 times the recommended dietary allowance for mice stimulated tumor growth by 164%.[124] There has been no research showing whether or not this effect occurs in humans.

General Prevention Data
Some studies have found associations between diets rich in thiamin and reduced rates of some forms of cancer. One of these studies found an association between increased dietary thiamin intake and reduced risk of colon cancer.[125]

Dosage and Toxicity:
For adults, the current dietary recommendations for thiamin are:
Men, age 19 and older: 1.2 milligrams
Women, age 19 and older: 1.1 milligrams
Pregnant women: 1.4 milligrams
Breastfeeding women: 1.5 milligrams
Thiamin has a low risk of toxicity. As a result, no upper level of intake for thiamin has been set. Individuals should note that the effect of high levels of thiamin intake upon tumor growth in humans has not been studied.

1 Prakash P, Krinsky NI, Russell RM. Retinoids, carotenoids, and human breast cancer cell cultures: a review of differential effects. Nutrition Review 2000; 58(6):170-6

2 Yang CC, Tu SF, Chang RC, Kao SY. In vitro cellular response of retinoic acid treated human oral cancer cell lines. Zhonghua Yi Xue Za Zhi (Taipei) 2001; 64(6):357 63.

3 Giacosa A, Filiberti R, Hill MJ, Faivre J. Vitamins and cancer chemoprevention. European Journal of Cancer Prevention 1997; 6 Suppl 1:S47-54.

4 Chen Y, Wu Q, Chen Z, Chen F, Su W. Effect of all-trans retinoic acid on growth of xenograft tumor and its metastatis in nude mice. Chinese Medical Journal 2000; 113(4):345-9.

5 Ponthan F, Borgstrom P, Hassan M, Wassberg E, Redfern CP, Kogner I. The vitamin A analogues: 13-cis retinoic acid, 9-cis retinoic acid, and Ro 13-6307 inhibit neuroblastoma tumour growth in vivo. Medical and Pediatric Oncology 2001; 36(1):127-31.

6 Chen Z, Wang Y, Wang W, Gong J, Xue Y. All-trans retinoic acid as a single agent induces complete remission in a patient with acute leukemia of M2a subtype. Chinese Medical Journal 2002; 115(1):58-61.

7 Egyed M, Mihalyfalvi Z, Kollar B, Rumi G, Keller E, Vass J, Fekete S. Effect of retinoic acid on the cytogenetic remission in the first chronic phase of chronic myeloid leukemia treated with interferon. Orvosi Hetilap (Hungary) 2001; 142(44):2421-5.

8 Visani G, et al. Pulsed ATRA as single therapy restores long-term remission in PML-RARalpha-positive acute promyelocytic leukemia patients in real time quantification of minimal residual disease. A pilot study. Leukemia 2001; 15(11):1696-700.

9 Hu J, Shen Z, Sun H, Wu W, Li X, Sun G, Wang Z. Long-term survey of outcome in acute promyelocytic leukemia. Chinese Medical Journal 2000; 113(2):107-10.

10 Mann G, Reinhardt D, Ritter J, et al. Treatment with all-trans retonic acid in acute promyelotic lukemia produces early deaths in children. Annals of Hematology 2001; 80(7):417-22.

11 Moon TE, Levine N, Cartmel B, Bangert JL, Rodney S, Dong Q, Peng YM, Alberts DS. Effect of retinol in preventing squamous cell skin cancer in moderate-risk subjects: a randomized, double-blind, controlled trial. Southwest Skin Cancer Prevention Study Group. Cancer, Epidemiology and Biomarkers Prevention 1997; 6(11):949-56.

12 van Zandwijk N, Dalesio O, Pastorino U, de Vries N, van Tinteren H. EUROSCAN, a randomized trial of vitamin A and N-acetylcysteine in patients with head and neck cancer or lung cancer. For the European Organization for Research and Treatment of Cancer Head and Neck and Lung Cancer Cooperative Groups. Journal of the National Cancer Institute 2000; 92(12):977-86.

13 Jyothirmayi R, Ramadas K, Varghese C, Jacob R, Nair MK, Sankaranarayanan R. Efficacy of vitamin A in the prevention of loco-regional recurrence and second primaries in head and neck cancer. European Journal of Cancer, Part B, Oral Oncology 1996; 32B(6):373-6.

14 Stich HF, Hornby AP, Mathew B, Sankaranarayanan R, Nair MK. Response of oral leukoplakias to the administration of vitamin A. Cancer Letters 1988; 40(1):93-101.

15 Roncucci L, Di Donato P, Carati L, Ferrari A, Perini M, Bertoni G, Bedogni G, Paris D, Svanoni F, Girola M, et al. Antioxidant vitamins or lactulose for the prevention of the recurrence of colorectal adenomas. Colorectal Cancer Study Group of the University of Modena and the Health Care District 16. Dis Colon Rectum. 1993; 36(3):227-34.

16 Omenn GS, Goodman GE, Thornquist MD, Balmes J, Cullen MR, Glass A, Keogh JP, Meyskens FL, Valanis B, Williams JH, Barnhart S, Hammar S. Effects of a combination of beta carotene and vitamin A on lung cancer and cardiovascular disease. New England Journal of Medicine 1996; 334(18):1150-5.

17 Zhang L, Zhai X, He Z. Modulating effect of vitamin D3 in vitro on EGFR mRNA expression of human breast cancer cell lines. Zhonghua Zhong Liu Za Zhi 2000; 22(3):205-7.

18 Diaz GD, Paraskeva C, Thomas MG, Binderup L, Hague A. Apoptosis is induced by the active metabolite of vitamin D3 and its analogue EB1089 in colorectal adenoma and carcinoma cells: possible implications for prevention and therapy. Cancer Research 2000; 60(8):2304-12.

[19] Liu W, Asa SL, Fantus IG, Walfish PG, Ezzat S. Vitamin D arrests thyroid carcinoma cell growth and induces p27 dephosphorylation and accumulation through PTEN/akt-dependent and –independent pathways. American Journal of Pathology 2002; 160(2):511-19.

[20] Prudencio J, et al. Action of low calcemic 1alpha,25-dihydroxyvitamin D3 analogue EB1089 in head and neck squamous cell carcinoma. Journal of the National Cancer Institute 2001; 93(10):745-53.

[21] Zhao XY, Feldman D. The role of vitamin D in prostate cancer. Steroids. 2001; 66(3-5): 293-300.

[22] Beer TM, Hough KM, Garzotto M, Lowe BA, Henner WD. Weekly high dose calcitriol and docetaxel in advanced prostate cancer. Seminars in Oncology 2001; 28(4 Suppl 15):49-55.

[23] Gross C, Stamey T, Hancock S, Feldman D. Treatment of early recurrent prostate cancer with 1,25-dihydroxyvitamin D3 (calcitriol). Journal of Urology 1998; 159(6):2035-9; discussion 2039-40.

[24] Osborn JL, Schwartz GG, Smith DC, Bahnson R, Day R, Trump, D. Phase II trial of oral 1,25 dihydroxyvitamin D (calcitriol) in hormone refractory prostate cancer. Urological Oncology 1995; 1(5):195-8.

[25] Zhao XY, Feldman D. The role of vitamin D in prostate cancer. Steroids 2001; 66(3-5): 293-300.

[26] Sung V, Feldman D. 1,25-dihydroxy-vitamin D3 decreases human prostate cancer cell adhesion and migration. Molecular and Cellular Endocrinology 2000; 164(1-2): 133-43.

[27] Masood R, et al. Kaposi sarcoma is a therapeutic target for vitamin D(3) receptor agonist. Blood 2000; 96(9):3188-94.

[28] Ferrero D, et al. Combined differentiating therapy for myelodysplastic syndromes: a phase II study. Leukemia Research 1996; 20(10):867-76.

[29] Lathers DM, Clark JI, Achille NJ, Young MR. Phase IB study of 25-hydroxyvitamin D(3) treatment to diminish suppressor cells in head and neck cancer patients. Human Immunology 2001; 62(11):1282-93.

[30] Nozoki T, et al. Effectiveness of activated vitamin D3 on improving prognosis of osteosarcoma patients. Oncology Reports 2001; 8(2):321-4.

[31] Trouillas P, Honnorat J, Bret P, Jouvet A, Gerard JP. Redifferentiation therapy in brain tumors: long-lasting complete regression of glioblastomas and an anaplastic astrocytoma under long term 1-alpha-hydroxycholecalciferol. Journal of Neurooncology 2001; 51(1):57-66.

[32] John EM, Schwartz GG, Dreon DM, Koo J. Vitamin D and breast cancer risk: the NHANES I epidemiologic follow-up study, 1971-1975 to 1992. National Health and Nutrition Examination Survey. Cancer Epidemiology, Biomarkers and Prevention 1999; 8(5):399-406.

[33] Janowsky EC, Lester GE, Weinberg CR, Millikan RC, Schildkraut JM, Garrett PA, Hulka BS. Association between low levels of 1,25-dihydroxyvitamin D and breast cancer risk. Public Health Nutrition 1999; 2(3):283-91.

[34] Garland CF, Garland FC, Gorham ED. Calcium and vitamin D. Their potential roles in colon and breast cancer prevention. Annals of the New York Academy of Sciences 1999; 889:107-19.

[35] Giovannucci E. Dietary influences of 1,25(OH)2 vitamin D in relation to prostate cancer: a hypothesis. Cancer Causes Control 1998; 9(6):567-82.

[36] Cameron E, Pauling L. Supplemental ascorbate in the supportive treatment of cancer: prolongation of survival times in terminal human cancer. Proceedings of the National Academy of Sciences USA 1976; 73(10):3685-9.

[37] Moertel CG, Fleming TR, Creagan ET, Rubin J, O'Connell MJ, Ames MM. High-dose vitamin C versus placebo in the treatment of patients with advanced cancer who have had no prior chemotherapy. A randomized double-blind comparison. New England Journal of Medicine 1985; 312(3): 137-41.

[38] Creagan ET, Moertel CG, O'Fallon JR, Schutt AJ, O'Connell MJ, Rubin J, Frytak S. Failure of high-dose vitamin C (ascorbic acid) therapy to benefit patients with advanced cancer. A controlled trial. New England Journal of Medicine 1979; 301(13):687-90.

[39] Padayatty SJ, Levine M. Reevaluation of ascorbate in cancer treatment: emerging evidence, open minds and serendipity. Journal of the American College of Nutrition 2000; 19(4):423-5.

40 Zhang ZW, Abdullahi M, Farthing MJ. Effect of physiological concentrations of vitamin C on gastric cancer cells and helicobacter pylori. Gut 2002; 50(2):165-9.

41 Vera JC, Rivas CI, Zhang RH, et al. Human HL-60 myeloid leukemia cells transport dehydroascorbic acid via the glucose transporters and accumulate reduced ascorbic acid. Blood 1994; 84(5):1628-34.

42 Akatov VS, et al. Combined vitamins B12b and C induce the glutathione depletion and the death of epidermoid human larynx carcinoma cells HEp-2. Bioscience Reports 2000; 20(5):411-7.

43 Bussey HJ, et al. A randomized trial of ascorbic acid in polyposis coli. Cancer 1982; 50(7):1434-9.

44 Barth TJ, et al. Redifferentiation of oral dysplastic mucosa by the application of the antioxidants beta-carotene, alpha-tocopherol, and vitamin C. International Journal for Vitamin and Nutrition Research 1997; 67(5):368-76.

45 McKeown-Eyssen G, Holloway C, Jazmaji V, Bright-See E, Dion P, Bruce WR. A randomized trial of vitamins C and E in the prevention of recurrence of colorectal polyps. Cancer Research 1988; 48(16):4701-5.

46 Correa P, Fontham ET, Bravo JC, Bravo LE, Ruiz B, Zarama G, Realpe JL, Malcom GT, Li D, Johnson WD, Mera R. Chemoprevention of gastric dysplasia: randomized trial of antioxidant supplements and antihelicobacter pylori therapy. Journal of the National Cancer Institute 2000; 92(23): 1881-8.

47 Cameron E, Campbell A. Innovation vs. quality control: an 'unpublishable' clinical trial of supplemental ascorbate in incurable cancer. Medical Hypotheses 1991; 36(3):185-9.

48 Murata A, Morishige F, Yamaguchi H. Prolongation of survival times of terminal cancer patients by administration of large doses of ascorbate. International Journal for Vitamin and Nutrition Research Supplement 1982; 23:103-13.

49 Carr AC, Frei B. Toward a new recommended dietary allowance for vitamin C based on antioxidant and health effects in humans. American Journal of Clinical Nutrition 1999; 69(6):1086-107.

50 Greenberg ER, Baron JA, Tosteson TD, Freeman DH Jr, Beck GJ, Bond JH,

Colacchio TA, Coller JA, Frankl HD, Haile RW, et al. A clinical trial of antioxidant vitamins to prevent colorectal adenoma. Polyp Prevention Study Group. New England Journal of Medicine 1994; 331(3):141-7.

51 Jacobs EJ, Connell CJ, Patel AV, Chao A, Rodriguez C, Seymour J, McCullough ML, Calle EE, Thun MJ. Vitamin C and vitamin E supplement use and colorectal cancer mortality in a large American Cancer Society cohort. Cancer Epidemiology, Biomarkers and Prevention 2001; 10(1):17-23.

52 Tannenbaum SR, Wishnok JS, Leaf CD. Inhibition of nitrosamine formation by ascorbic acid. American Journal of Clinical Nutrition 1991; 53(1 Suppl):247S-250S.

53 Blot WJ, Li JY, Taylor PR, Guo W, Dawsey S, Wang GQ, Yang CS, Zheng SF, Gail M, Li GY, et al. Nutrition intervention trials in Linxian, China: supplementation with specific vitamin/mineral combinations, cancer incidence, and disease-specific mortality in the general population. Journal of the National Cancer Institute 1993; 85(18):1483-92.

54 Palozza P, et al. Beta-carotene at high concentrations induces apoptosis by enhancing oxy-radical production in human adenocarcinoma lines. Free Radical Biology and Medicine 2001; 30(9):1000-7.

55 Zhu Y, Hao X, Sun H. Effect of beta-carotene on mouse transplantable mammary cancer MA737. Zhonghua Zhong Liu Za Zhi 1999; 21(4):262-4.

56 Mayne ST, Cartmel B, Baum M, Shor-Posner G, Fallon BG, Briskin K, Bean J, Zheng T, Cooper D, Friedman C, Goodwin WJ Jr. Randomized trial of supplemental beta-carotene to prevent second head and neck cancer. Cancer Research 2001; 61(4):1457-63.

57 Greenberg ER, Baron JA, Stukel TA, Stevens MM, Mandel JS, Spencer SK, Elias PM, Lowe N, Nierenberg DW, Bayrd G, et al. A clinical trial of beta carotene to prevent basal-cell and squamous-cell cancers of the skin. The Skin Cancer Prevention Study Group. New England Journal of Medicine 1990; 323(12):789-95.

58 Garewal HS, et al. Beta-carotene produces sustained remissions in patients with oral leukoplakia: results of a multicenter prospective trial. Archives of Otolaryngology - Head and Neck Surgery 1999; 125(12):1305-10.

[59] Greenwald P, Clifford CK, Milner JA. Diet and cancer prevention. European Journal of Cancer 2001; 37(8):948-65.

[60] Lee IM, Cook NR, Manson JE, Buring JE, Hennekens CH. Beta-carotene supplementation and incidence of cancer and cardiovascular disease: the Women's Health Study. Journal of the National Cancer Institute 1999; 91(24):2102-6.

[61] Hennekens CH, Buring JE, Manson JE, Stampfer M, Rosner B, Cook NR, Belanger C, LaMotte F, Gaziano JM, Ridker PM, Willett W, Peto R. Lack of effect of long-term supplementation with beta carotene on the incidence of malignant neoplasms and cardiovascular disease. New England Journal of Medicine 1996; 334(18):1145-9.

[62] Green A, Williams G, Neale R, Hart V, Leslie D, Parsons P, Marks GC, Gaffney P, Battistutta D, Frost C, Lang C, Russell A. Daily sunscreen application and beta carotene supplementation in prevention of basal cell and squamous cell carcinomas of the skin: a randomised controlled trial. Lancet 1999; 354(9180):723-9.

[63] The Alpha-Tocopherol, Beta Carotene Cancer Prevention Study Group. The effect of vitamin E and beta carotene on the incidence of lung cancer and other cancers in male smokers. New England Journal of Medicine 1994; 330(15):1029-35.

[64] Heinonen OP, Albanes D, Virtamo J, Taylor PR, Huttunen JK, Hartman AM, Haapakoski J, Malila N, Rautalahti M, Ripatti S, Maenpaa H, Teerenhovi L, Koss L, Virolainen M, Edwards BK. Prostate cancer and supplementation with alpha-tocopherol and beta-carotene: incidence and mortality in a controlled trial. Journal of the National Cancer Institute 1998; 90(6):440-6.

[65] Redman C, Scott JA, Baines AT, Basye JL, Clark LC, Calley C, Roe D, Payne CM, Nelson MA. Inhibitory effect of selenomethionine on the growth of three selected human tumor cell lines. Cancer Letters 1998; 125(1-2):103-10.

[66] Ip C. Prophylaxis of mammary neoplasia by selenium supplementation in the initiation and promotion phases of chemical carcinogenesis. Cancer Research 1981; 41(11 Pt 1):4386-90.

[67] Thirunavukkarasu C, Singh JP, Selvendiran K, Sakthisekaran D. Chemopreventive efficacy of selenium against N-nitrosodiethylamine-induced hepatoma in albino rats. Cell Biochemistry and Function 2001; 19:265-71.

[68] Pakdaman A. Symptomatic treatment of brain tumor patients with sodium selenite, oxygen, and other supportive measures. Biological Trace Element Research 1998; 62:1-6.

[69] Lockwood K, Moesgaard S, Hanioka T, Folkers K. Apparent partial remission of breast cancer in 'high risk' patients supplemented with nutritional antioxidants, essential fatty acids, and coenzyme Q10. Molecular Aspects of Medicine 1994; 15: 231-40.

[70] Toma S, et al. Selenium therapy in patients with precancerous and malignant oral cavity lesions: preliminary results. Cancer Detection and Prevention 1991; 15:491-4.

[71] Combs GF Jr, Clark LC, Turnbull BW. Reduction of cancer mortality and incidence by selenium supplementation. Medizinische Klinik 1997; 92 Suppl 3:42-5.

[72] Yoshizawa K, Willett WC, Morris SJ, Stampfer MJ, Spiegelman D, Rimm EB, Giovannucci E. Study of prediagnostic selenium level in toenails and the risk of advanced prostate cancer. Journal of the National Cancer Institute 1998; 90(16):1219-24.

[73] Brooks JD, Metter EJ, Chan DW, Sokoll LJ, Landis P, Nelson WG, Muller D, Andres R, Carter HB. Plasma selenium level before diagnosis and the risk of prostate cancer development. Journal of Urology 2001; 166(6):2034-8.

[74] Ghadirian P, Maisonneuve P, Perret C, Kennedy G, Boyle P, Krewski D, Lacroix A. A case-control study of toenail selenium and cancer of the breast, colon, and prostate. Cancer Detection and Prevention 2000; 24(4):305-13.

[75] Garland M, Morris JS, Stampfer MJ, Colditz GA, Spate VL, Baskett CK, Rosner B, Speizer FE, Willett WC, Hunter DJ. Prospective study of toenail selenium levels and cancer among women. Journal of the National Cancer Institute 1995; 87(7):497-505.

[76] Hunter DJ, Morris JS, Stampfer MJ, Colditz GA, Speizer FE, Willett WC. A prospective study of selenium status and breast cancer risk. Journal of the American Medical Association 1990; 264(9):1128-31.

[77] Yu SY, Zhu YJ, Li WG. Protective role of selenium against hepatitis B virus and primary liver cancer in Qidong. Biological Trace Element Research 1997; 56(1):117-24.

[78] Li W, Zhu Y, Yan X, et al. The prevention of primary liver cancer by selenium in high risk populations. Zhonghua Yu Fang Yi Xue Za Zhi. 2000; 34(6):336-8.

[79] National Cancer Institute. Largest-ever prostate cancer prevention trial opens: 32,000 men sought to test vitamin E and selenium. NIH News Release. http://www.nih.gov/news/pr/jul2001/nci-24.htm.

[80] Fleshner NE, Kucuk O. Antioxidant dietary supplements: Rationale and current status as chemopreventive agents for prostate cancer. Urology 2001; 57(4 Suppl 1):90-4.

[81] Nesaretnam K, Dorasamy S, Darbre PD. Tocotrienols inhibit growth of ZR-75-1 breast cancer cells. International Journal of Food Science Nutrition 2000; 51 Suppl:S95-103.

[82] Israel K, Yu W, Sanders BG, Kline K. Vitamin E succinate induces apoptosis in human prostate cancer cells: role for Fas in vitamin E succinate-triggered apoptosis. Nutrition and Cancer 2000; 36(1):90-100.

[83] Gunawardena K, Murray DK, Meikle AW. Vitamin E and other antioxidants inhibit human prostate cancer cells through apoptosis. Prostate 2000; 44(4):287-95.

[84] Neuzil J, Weber T, Terman A, Weber C, Brunk UT. Vitamin E analogues as inducers of apoptosis: implications for their potential antineoplastic role. Redox Report 2001; 6:143-51.

[85] Gogos CA, et al. Dietary omega-3 polyunsaturated fatty acids plus vitamin E restore immunodeficiency and prolong survival for severely ill patients with generalized malignancy: a randomized control trial. Cancer 1998; 82:395-402.

[86] Schwenke DC. Does lack of tocopherols and tocotrienols put women at increased risk of breast cancer? Journal of Nutritional Biochemistry 2002; 13(1):2-20.

[87] Voorrips LE, Goldbohm RA, Brants HA, van Poppel GA, Sturmans F, Hermus RJ, van den Brandt PA. A prospective cohort study on antioxidant and folate intake and male lung cancer risk. Cancer Epidemiology, Biomarkers and Prevention 2000; 9(4):357-65.

[88] Bostick RM, Potter JD, McKenzie DR, Sellers TA, Kushi LH, Steinmetz KA, Folsom AR. Reduced risk of colon cancer with high intake of vitamin E: the Iowa Women's Health Study. Cancer Research 1993; 53(18):4230-7.

[89] Slattery ML, Edwards SL, Anderson K, Caan B. Vitamin E and colon cancer: is there an association? Nutrition and Cancer 1998; 30(3):201-6.

[90] Albanes D, Malila N, Taylor PR, Huttunen JK, Virtamo J, Edwards BK, Rautalahti M, Hartman AM, Barrett MJ, Pietinen P, Hartman TJ, Sipponen P, Lewin K, Teerenhovi L, Hietanen P, Tangrea JA, Virtanen M, Heinonen OP. Effects of supplemental alpha-tocopherol and beta-carotene on colorectal cancer: results from a controlled trial (Finland). Cancer Causes Control 2000; 11(3):197-205.

[91] McLaughlin JK, Gridley G, Block G, Winn DM, Preston-Martin S, Schoenberg JB, Greenberg RS, Stemhagen A, Austin DF, Ershow AG, et al. Dietary factors in oral and pharyngeal cancer. Journal of the National Cancer Institute 1988; 80(15):1237-43.

[92] Gridley G, McLaughlin JK, Block G, Blot WJ, Gluch M, Fraumeni JF Jr. Vitamin supplement use and reduced risk of oral and pharyngeal cancer. American Journal of Epidemiology 1992; 135(10):1083-92.

[93] Barone J, Taioli E, Hebert JR, Wynder EL. Vitamin supplement use and risk for oral and esophageal cancer. Nutrition and Cancer 1992; 18(1):31-41.

[94] Mayne ST, Risch HA, Dubrow R, Chow WH, Gammon MD, Vaughan TL, Farrow DC, Schoenberg JB, Stanford JL, Ahsan H, West AB, Rotterdam H, Blot WJ, Fraumeni JF Jr. Nutrient intake and risk of subtypes of esophageal and gastric cancer. Cancer Epidemiology, Biomarkers and Prevention 2001; 10:1055-62.

[95] Michaud DS, Spiegelman D, Clinton SK, Rimm EB, Willett WC, Giovannucci E. Prospective study of dietary supplements, macronutrients, micronutrients, and risk of bladder cancer in US men. American Journal of Epidemiology 2000; 152(12):1145-53.

[96] Zeegers MP, Goldbohm RA, van den Brandt PA. Are retinol, vitamin C, vitamin E, folate and carotenoids intake associated with bladder cancer risk? Results from the Netherlands Cohort Study. British Journal of Cancer 2001; 85(7):977-83.

[97] Slattery ML, Abbott TM, Overall JC Jr, Robison LM, French TK, Jolles C, Gardner JW, West DW. Dietary vitamins A, C, and E and selenium as risk factors for cervical cancer. Epidemiology 1990; 1(1):8-15.

[98] Potischman N, Herrero R, Brinton LA, Reeves WC, Stacewicz-Sapuntzakis M, Jones CJ, Brenes MM, Tenorio F, de Britton RC, Gaitan E. A case-control study of nutrient status and invasive cervical cancer. II. Serologic indicators. American Journal of Epidemiology 1991; 134(11):1347-55.

[99] McCann SE, Moysich KB, Mettlin C. Intakes of selected nutrients and food groups and risk of ovarian cancer. Nutrition and Cancer 2001; 39(1):19-28.

[100] Fairfield KM, Hankinson SE, Rosner BA, Hunter DJ, Colditz GA, Willett WC. Risk of ovarian carcinoma and consumption of vitamins A, C, and E and specific carotenoids: a prospective analysis. Cancer 2001; 92(9):2318-26.

[101] Burney PG, Comstock GW, Morris JS. Serologic precursors of cancer: serum micronutrients and the subsequent risk of pancreatic cancer. American Journal of Clinical Nutrition 1989; 49(5):895-900.

[102] Rautalahti MT, Virtamo JR, Taylor PR, Heinonen OP, Albanes D, Haukka JK, Edwards BK, Karkkainen PA, Stolzenberg-Solomon RZ, Huttunen J. The effects of supplementation with alpha-tocopherol and beta-carotene on the incidence and mortality of carcinoma of the pancreas in a randomized, controlled trial. Cancer 1999; 86(1): 37-42.

[103] Bunk MN, Dnistrian AM, Schwartz MK, et al. Dietary zinc deficiency decreases plasma concentrations of vitamin E. Proceedings of the Society of Experimental and Biological Medicine 1989; 190:379-84.

[104] Baron JA, Beach M, Mandel JS, van Stolk RU, Haile RW, Sandler RS, Rothstein R, Summers RW, Snover DC, Beck GJ, Bond JH, Greenberg ER. Calcium supplements for the prevention of colorectal adenomas. Calcium Polyp Prevention Study Group. New England Journal of Medicine 1999; 340(2): 101-7.

[105] Bonithon-Kopp C, Kronborg O, Giacosa A, Rath U, Faivre J. Calcium and fibre supplementation in prevention of colorectal adenoma recurrence: a randomised intervention trial. European Cancer Prevention Organisation Study Group. Lancet 2000; 356(9238):1300-6.

[106] Cascinu S, Ligi M, Del Ferro E, Foglietti G, Cioccolini P, Staccioli MP, Carnevali A, Luigi Rocchi MB, Alessandroni P, Giordani P, Catalano V, Polizzi V, Agostinelli R, Muretto P, Catalano G. Effects of calcium and vitamin supplementation on colon cell proliferation in colorectal cancer. Cancer Investigations 2000; 18(5):411-6.

[107] Lipkin M. Preclinical and early human studies of calcium and colon cancer prevention. Annals of the New York Acadamy of Science 1999; 889:120-7.

[108] Chan JM, Stampfer MJ, Ma J, Gann PH, Gaziano JM, Giovannucci EL. Dairy products, calcium, and prostate cancer risk in the Physicians' Health Study. American Journal of Clinical Nutrition 2001; 74(4):549-54.

[109] Tavani A, Gallus S, Franceschi S, La Vecchia C. Calcium, dairy products, and the risk of prostate cancer. Prostate 2001; 48(2): 118-21.

[110] Kim YI, et al. Effects of folate supplementation on two provisional molecular markers of colon cancer: a prospective, randomized trial. American Journal of Gastroenterology 2001; 96:184-95.

[111] Butterworth CE Jr., et al. Improvement in cervical dysplasia associated with folic acid therapy in users of oral contraceptives. American Journal of Clinical Nutrition 1982; 35:73-82.

[112] Potischman N, Briton LA. Nutrition and cervical neoplasia. Cancer Causes and Control 1996; 7:113-26.

[113] Butterworth CE Jr. Folate status, women's health, pregnancy outcome, and cancer. Journal of the American College of Nutrition 1993; 12:438-41.

[114] Harper JM, et al. Erythrocyte folate levels, oral contraceptive use and abnormal cervical cytology. Acta Cytologica 1994; 38:324-30.

[115] Grio R, et al. Antineoblastic activity of antioxidant vitamins: the role of folic acid in the prevention of cervical dysplasia. Panminerva Medica 1993; 35:193-6.

[116] Kiu T, et al. A longitudinal analysis of human papillomavirus 16 infection, nutritional status, and cervical dysplasia progression. Cancer Epidemiology, Biomarkers and Prevention 1995; 4:373-80.

117 Eichholzer M, Luthy J, Moser U, Fowler B. Folate and the risk of colorectal, breast and cervix cancer: the epidemiological evidence. Swiss Medical Weekly 2001; 131(37-38):539-49.

118 Giovannucci E, Stampfer MJ, Colditz GA, Hunter DJ, Fuchs C, Rosner BA, Speizer FE, Willett WC. Multivitamin use, folate, and colon cancer in women in the Nurses' Health Study. Annals of Internal Medicine 1998; 129(7):517-24.

119 Zhang S, Hunter DJ, Hankinson SE, Giovannucci EL, Rosner BA, Colditz GA, Speizer FE, Willett WC. A prospective study of folate intake and the risk of breast cancer. Journal of the American Medical Association 1999; 281(17):1632-7.

120 Shrubsole MJ, Jin F, Dai Q, Shu XO, Potter JD, Hebert JR, Gao YT, Zheng W. Dietary folate intake and breast cancer risk: results from the Shanghai Breast Cancer Study. Cancer Research 2001; 61(19):7136-41.

121 Nelson RL. Iron and colorectal cancer risk: human studies. Nutrition Reviews 2001; 59(5):140-8.

122 Wurzelmann JI, Silver A, Schreinemachers DM, Sandler RS, Everson RB. Iron intake and the risk of colorectal cancer. Cancer Epidemiology, Biomarkers and Prevention 1996; 5(7):503-7.

123 Boros LG, Brandes JL, Lee WN, Cascante M, Puigjaner J, Revesz E, Bray TM, Schirmer WJ, Melvin WS. Thiamine supplementation to cancer patients: a double edged sword. Anticancer Research 1998; 18(1B): 595-602.

124 Comin-Anduix B, Boren J, Martinez S, Moro C, Centelles JJ, Trebukhina R, Petushok N, Lee WN, Boros LG, Cascante M. The effect of thiamine supplementation on tumour proliferation. A metabolic control analysis study. European Journal of Biochemistry 2001; 268(15):4177-82.

125 Slattery ML, Potter JD, Coates A, Ma KN, Berry TD, Duncan DM, Caan BJ. Plant foods and colon cancer: an assessment of specific foods and their related nutrients. Cancer Causes Control 1997; 8(4):575-90.

Chapter Five

Herbals

It is often difficult to be sure that over-the-counter herbal and botanical supplements contain the ingredients they claim. The 1994 Dietary Supplements and Health Education Act established a framework for FDA regulation of manufacturing practices, instituted an Office of Dietary Supplement Research at NIH, and funded four university-based centers for Dietary Supplement Research in Botanicals. However, no regulatory body exists to verify the claims of every supplement manufacturer.

It is vitally important to inform your health professional about each of the herbal or botanical supplements you are taking, because these substances can interfere with the actions of cancer drugs.

Some recently designed and marketed supplements are not derived from plant sources at all, but are included in this chapter because they are popularly considered "herbal supplements" and sold alongside herbals and botanicals.

MISTLETOE

Mistletoe extracts have been proposed for the treatment of cancer since the early part of the twentieth century. Iscador is a commercially available extract of the mistletoe plant, and the extract used in most of the clinical studies.

Evidence:

In vitro and animal studies have not as yet identified the most important mechanism of action or constituent of mistletoe. Some studies have indicated an immune stimulatory effect of compounds known as lectins,[1] while other studies have shown direct cancer cell-killing effects of mistletoe alkaloids and viscotoxins.[2,3] A laboratory study involving human liver cancer cells found that Korean mistletoe lectin reduced the proliferation of these cancer cells and increased the amount of apoptosis in the cell population.[4] A different study found that mistletoe extracts enhanced the ability of a variety of anticancer agents to destroy lung cancer cells.[5]

A case report of a 44-year-old man with follicular non-Hodgkin's lymphoma suggested that treatment with Iscador led to complete regional remission and improved quality-of-life in the patient.[6] Cessation of mistletoe therapy led to disease progression, whereas the resumption of therapy again led to disease remission. The patient had been successfully treated over a 12-year-period. A clinical trial found that Iscador administration to patients who had been previously treated with surgery for pulmonary cancer led to increased survival time compared to a control group.[7]

Several clinical trials have analyzed the effectiveness of Iscador in the treatment of various tumor types. In one study, 1,600 patients who had undergone treatment with Iscador were compared to 8,400 patients receiving standard therapy for a variety of different tumor types. Patients who received Iscador treatment lived on average 40% longer than control group patients.[8]

In a separate study, patients with stage III or IV gliomas (a type of malignant brain tumor) treated with mistletoe extract had greater than double overall survival time compared to patients not receiving treatment.[9] A study of 8 breast cancer patients found that 16 weeks of therapy with mistletoe extract led to immune system changes that are unfavorable to tumor growth.[10] A study of 20 cancer patients who had evidence of malignant cells in their plural fluid found that the administration of the mistletoe extract Helixor reduced the number of malignant cells by 72%.[11]

A retrospective review of incurable stomach cancer cases found that mistletoe administration produced slightly increased survival times and a greater percentage of patients who survived to the two-year-point.[12] A study involving 7 cancer patients with pleural carcinomatosis found that 1 ml of 5% Iscador led to a "marked" reduction in tumor size.[13] A retrospective review of 69 cases of distant cancers that had metastasized to the liver found that Helixor increased survival time by more than three-fold compared to a control group.[14]

No objective responses to mistletoe therapy were seen in patients with advanced cancers of the pancreas[15] or kidneys.[16]

Data presented in 1999 at a European cancer conference showed Iscador to be ineffective in prevention of recurrence of melanoma after surgery.[17]

Dosage and Toxicity:

Mistletoe extracts are generally administered subcutaneously several times per week on an experimental basis. Adverse effects of mistletoe are rare, with local inflammatory responses being the most commonly reported reaction.[18] Past clinical trials have involved daily doses of 10 g drug. Whole mistletoe is extremely toxic, and overdose can be fatal.

CORIOLUS VERSICOLOR

Coriolus versicolor, also known as the cloud mushroom, was used to treat people with cancer in Traditional Japanese Medicine. There are several different commercially available extracts of Coriolus mushrooms, the most commonly used medically being PSP and PSK.

Evidence:

Evidence from several laboratory studies has supported the idea that Coriolus stimulates the immune system, specifically T and B lymphocytes, as well as natural killer cells.[19] There is also growing evidence that the active constituents of Coriolus are the protein-bound polysaccharides.[20]

A study involving mice found that the administration of PSP reduced the size of brain tumors in the treated animals compared to controls.[21] An additional study in mice found that PSP can slow the progression of tumors caused by herpes virus infections by its strong toxic effects on cancer cells.[22] Other research has found evidence that PSK suppresses cancer metastasis in mice and rats and suppresses the metastasis of human lung and prostate cancer metastasis in laboratory studies.[23]

A smaller protein derived from Coriolus versicolor called SPCV has been found to have potent toxic effects on a variety of human cancer cell lines.[24] In some cases, these effects were much greater than with the PSP and PSK types. A laboratory study involving human prostate cancer cell lines found that Coriolus versicolor extracts decreased cancer cell growth in cells that are responsive to male hormones.[25]

A number of clinical studies have analyzed the effectiveness of PSK as an adjunct to conventional therapeutics. Addition of PSK to radiation therapy for non-small cell lung cancer significantly improved five-year survival in one clinical trial.[26] When PSK was added to chemotherapy after surgery for stomach cancer, five-year survival improved from 60 to 73%.[27]

In patients who had undergone surgery to remove colorectal cancers, PSK administration without any other conventional treatment significantly improved five-year survival rates.[28] Oral administration of PSK was able to significantly improve survival and lengthen remissions in patients with acute leukemias (both AML and ALL).[29] A prospective controlled trial for lung cancer patients who had received radiation found that PSK combined with chemotherapy produced significantly longer disease-free intervals and survival rates than with chemotherapy alone.[30]

A prospective study in patients with nasopharyngeal cancer reported longer survival periods compared to historical controls.[31] Two of three randomized controlled trials involving patients with esophageal cancer found significantly better survival times in the groups treated with PSK.[32,33] An additional randomized controlled trial found improved immune system effects in gastric and colon cancer patients who had received PSK.[34] A randomized controlled trial of 73 leukemia patients found that PSK treatment produced a significant extension of remission and survival at a follow-up analysis at 6 months.[35]

No significant survival benefit was seen when PSK was used in addition to chemotherapy after surgery for patients with breast cancer.[36]

Dosage and Toxicity:

The usual dose of PSK in these clinical trials was 3 grams per day. Although studies have not compared the difference between short-term dosing and long-term dosing, PSK researchers suggest that this treatment needs to be continued for a period of years to show a benefit. Side effects with PSK have been mild, and include changes in the color of the nails and coughing.

GINSENG

There are three different herbs commonly referred to as ginseng: Asian ginseng (Panax ginseng), Siberian ginseng (Eleutherococcus senticosus) and American ginseng (Panax quinquefolius). While there are subtle differences in the historical uses of these herbs, each has been used as a tonic. Tonic herbs are used to treat people who are debilitated, fatigued or have difficulty responding to stress. Both Asian and Siberian ginseng are among the most commonly used herbal products in the world.

Evidence:

Ginseng products have been used in Traditional Chinese Medicine for both cancer prevention and treatment. A study in rats found that a diet containing 1% Panax ginseng given for a period of five weeks inhibited the development of colon cancer compared to a control group.[37] A study involving mice found that Panax ginseng given in doses of 400 mg/kg of body weight significantly inhibited mouse sarcoma and melanoma tumor development.[38]

Chemicals common to all ginseng products have been studied *in vitro*, and were found to inhibit the growth of various cancer cell lines.[39] A study of human ovarian cancer cells *in vitro* and *in vivo* found that extracts of Panax ginseng had additive anti-cancer effects when combined with other chemotherapy agents.[40] A different *in vitro* study found that a metabolite of ginseng inhibited the proliferation of human leukemia, pulmonary adenocarcinoma and hepatoma cells.[41] Although the concentrations necessary to produce such inhibition were higher than those required of cisplatin, a commonly-used chemotherapy agent, the researchers concluded that these ginseng extracts had great potential as a therapeutic agent for these types of cancer.

Some,[42,43] but not all,[44] studies have found ginseng extracts to stimulate immune function in healthy people. Formulas containing Asian ginseng (along with other herbs) have been reported in studies from China and Japan to reduce side effects and improve the efficacy of chemotherapy agents.[45-47] These studies did not include control groups. No controlled studies have yet been published on the effect of Asian ginseng alone in patients with cancer.

In patients undergoing surgical treatment of cancer, supplementation with Siberian ginseng was shown to reduce surgical complications, shorten duration of hospital stay, and reduce surgical mortality compared to a control group.[48]

A preliminary study from Russia concluded that Siberian ginseng stimulated function of the immune system in patients undergoing chemotherapy and radiation treatment for breast cancer.[49]

No studies have analyzed the effect of American ginseng in patients with cancer.

Dosage and Toxicity:

Asian ginseng is often taken as a standardized herbal extract, at doses of 100-200 mg per day. Alcohol tincture taken at ½ tsp three times per day can be used as well. For Siberian ginseng, a widely recommended dose is 2-3 grams of whole herb or 2 tsp of alcohol tincture per day.

All three forms of ginseng are generally considered to have low potential for toxicity at recommended doses. Individuals who are trying to keep their blood pressure under control should be aware that high doses of ginseng have been shown to increase blood pressure. Because of possible drug/herb interactions, use of ginseng is not recommended for individuals taking Coumadin, warfarin or digoxin. Ginseng may also impede the efficacy of other drugs, so check with your health professional. Little is known about the potential for positive or negative interactions between conventional chemotherapy and ginseng of any type.

CURCUMIN

Curcumin is a component of the turmeric plant. It is an important herb in the traditional medical system of India, known as Ayurvedic Medicine. Standardized botanical extracts of curcumin are now widely available in America.

Evidence:

Several laboratory and clinical studies have investigated multiple mechanisms of action by which curcumin may exert anticancer activity.

Curcumin is thought to exert anti-inflammatory effects by blocking an enzyme called COX-2.[50] (Pharmaceutical drugs that block this enzyme have been studied as potential cancer fighting treatments.[51]) In one double-blind clinical trial, curcumin was found to have superior anti-inflammatory activity to placebo and a standard non-steroidal medication.[52]

Laboratory studies have also shown curcumin to be a potent antioxidant.[53] This antioxidant action may be responsible for the documented ability of curcumin to block cancer progression in animal experiments.[54]

A study involving human melanoma cell lines found that curcumin can induce apoptosis, or cell death, in eight types of melanoma cell lines.[55] Yet another study found that curcumin induced apoptosis in human basal cell carcinoma cells.[56]

A different study involving human prostate cells transplanted into mice found that a diet containing 2% curcumin reduced the proliferation of cells and increased the amount of apoptosis.[57] In a different study involving mice, researchers found that animals fed a diet containing 0.2% curcumin were 81% less likely to develop liver tumors compared to control animals.[58] All of the animals were exposed to an agent known to induce liver cancer in mice.

In one preliminary clinical trial, oral administration of curcumin led to histological improvement in precancerous conditions in 7 of 25 patients.[59] Beneficial effects were also seen in lesions in the cervix, stomach, bladder and oral cavity.

In patients with advanced colon cancer refractory to conventional treatment, administration of up to 180 mg per day of curcumin led to disease stabilization for 2 to 4 months in 5 of 15 patients.[60] This study has not yet been followed up with larger clinical trials.

Dosage and Toxicity:

The maximum tolerated dose of curcumin in a Phase I clinical trial was 8,000 mg per day.[61] No toxicity was reported up to this dosage level. Above this level, the bulky volume of the drug was unacceptable to patients.

At the 8,000 mg dose, but not at doses of 180 mg per day,[62] curcumin is measurable in the blood stream.

ASTRAGALUS

Astragalus is an herb that has been used for thousands of years in Traditional Chinese Medicine (TCM). The TCM use of this herb has largely been as an immune stimulating agent.

Evidence:

Animal research has suggested the ability of Astragalus extracts to influence the actions of the immune system,[63] and a similar immune-stimulating response has also been documented in humans, at least in patients with compromised immune function.[64] A study of healthy and cancerous blood cells obtained from patients and treated in the laboratory with Astragalus found that this herb stimulated immune factors that killed the cancerous cells.[65] A different study found that Astragalus increased the ability of chemotherapeutic drugs to kill melanoma cells in the body.[66] An additional study verified this finding.[67]

TCM formulas containing Astragalus in combination with other herbs have also been found to maintain white blood cell counts in patients undergoing cancer treatment.[68, 69] Low white blood cell counts are common during chemotherapy and can lead to serious infections. A case report involving a person with carcinoma of the lung found that the administration of 15 grams per day of the Chinese medicine called Ren-Shen-Yang-Rong-Tang for 7 weeks led to decreased levels of tumor marker.[70] This formulation contains Astragalus and 11 other crude natural substances.

The effect of Astragalus as a primary treatment for cancer has not been tested in modern clinical trials. Also, the effect of Astragalus on the therapeutic action of chemotherapy agents has not been studied.

Dosage and Toxicity:
Most herbal texts suggest 3-6 grams per day of encapsulated whole herb or 2-3 tsp of alcohol tincture per day.

CAT'S CLAW

Cat's claw (also referred to as una da gato) is an herb used in Traditional Peruvian Medicine. It was used as an anti-inflammatory agent, and perhaps in the treatment of tumors as well. Cat's claw is relatively new to the United States, only gaining popularity in the last 20 years.

Evidence:
There are a number of mechanisms by which cat's claw could potentially be useful for patients with cancer. Extracts of the herb have been found to be anti-inflammatory in people with arthritis.[71] The anti-inflammatory action of cat's claw was at least partially mediated by the blocking of particular signaling molecules (TNF alpha and prostaglandin E2) thought to cause some of the systemic ill effects of advanced cancers.

In another study, cat's claw was found to raise white blood cell levels in healthy people.[72] Low white blood cell counts are another common problem in patients with advanced cancers.

In vitro studies have shown a direct toxic effect of cat's claw on breast cancer cells,[73] although it is not known if cat's claw would have a similar effect at blood concentrations achievable by oral doses of the herb.

An unpublished case report of 3 patients with metastatic colon or ovarian cancer found that 2 of the patients had no evidence of cancer and the other patient had a smaller tumor after evaluation at 4 and 7 months.[74] These patients had previously received conventional therapy. Two clinic series, with 22 and 78 patients respectively, conducted in Europe found benefits in all patients who received cat's claw.[75] A total of 19 of 22 patients in the first series and all of the patients in the second series received conventional therapy initially.

No human studies have assessed cat's claw, either alone or with conventional medicines, as a treatment for cancer.

Dosage and Toxicity:
The usual dosage of cat's claw used for anti-inflammatory purposes is $\frac{1}{4}$-$\frac{1}{2}$ tsp of cat's claw alcohol tincture twice per day. The safety of cat's claw has been established in Phase I clinical trials with healthy people,[76] but not in patients with cancer.

MODIFIED CITRUS PECTIN

Modified citrus pectin (MCP) is a complex sugar molecule found in the peel or pulp of citrus fruits. It is modified by heat and pH changes to split the molecule into smaller and more absorbable short-chain pectins. MCP is also sometimes referred to as fractionated pectin.

Evidence:
Cell-surface receptors known as galactin-3 molecules are thought to be necessary to allow cancer cells to spread to other organs, a process known as metastasis. Evidence from *in vitro* studies with citrus pectin have identified at least one possible mechanism by which MCP may influence the spread of cancer: MCP may block the ability of galactin-3 sites on cancer cells to bind to vessel walls, which would in turn inhibit blood-borne metastasis, or possibly inhibit new blood vessel formation.[77]

In fact, MCP has been shown to inhibit metastasis of melanoma[78] and prostate tumors[77] in animal studies. In the melanoma study, MCP was given as an injection, while in the prostate tumor study, MCP was administered orally.

One animal study showed up to 70% shrinkage in colon tumors in animals treated with oral MCP.[79] A different study in rats found that animals fed a diet containing 15% MCP led to metabolic changes that increased apoptosis, or cell death, in colon cancer cells.[80] A study in mice found that MCP given in doses of either 0.8 mg or 1.6 mg per milliliter of water reduced the growth of solid primary tumors.[79]

An *in vitro* study of human prostate cancer cells found that MCP decreased the proliferation of cancer cells by modifying a key protein in the proliferation process.[81] In a preliminary study of prostate cancer patients whose cancers had progressed on conventional treatment, oral MCP slowed the amount of time it took for PSA levels to double in four of seven patients.[82] PSA doubling time is a surrogate blood measurement of disease activity.

Dosage and safety:

MCP has not yet undergone a Phase I (dose-finding) study, so the optimal dose of MCP has yet to be determined. The only published human study of the effect of MCP used a dose of 5 grams, three times daily.

No adverse effects of MCP administration have been noted in the animal or human studies of this compound.

PC-SPES

PC-SPES is a proprietary formula marketed for the treatment of prostate cancer. The herbs contained in the formula are Isatis indigotica, Glycyrrhiza glabra, Panax pseudoginseng, Ganoderma lucidum, Scutellaria baicalensis, Dendrantherma morifolium, Serenoa repens, and Robdosia rubescens. There has been suggestion in the research literature that there are additional non-herbal constituents in PC-SPES. **This has led to a voluntary product recall, which remains in place as this book goes to press.**

Although it is debated whether PC-SPES actually contains added estrogenic compounds, the herbs in the formula clearly have estrogenic effect. This may be the major reason for the clinical benefits seen with PC-SPES. Also, a number of these herbs have been used in Traditional Chinese Medicine to treat different cancer types. Given this pattern of traditional use, it is possible that there are other benefits of these herbs, as well.

Evidence:

A substance called baicalin, a significant component of PC-SPES has been found to inhibit human cancer cell proliferation using apoptotic and cell cycle arrest mechanisms.[83] Studies have provided evidence that human prostate cancer cells transplanted into mice are inhibited both *in vivo* and *in vitro* when exposed to PC-SPES.[84]

A report of 4 cases of advanced prostate carcinoma found that prostate antigen (PSA) levels rose rapidly after PC-SPES was discontinued.[85] PSA is a commonly used marker for prostate cancer. An additional case study involving two cases of prostate cancer, which had not responded to previous therapy, found that PC-SPES has significant estrogen activity and produced a more than three-fold decrease in PSA levels in these 2 patients after 1 and 4 months.[86]

A study of 69 patients with prostate cancer found that cancer cells were inhibited through apoptosis both *in vitro* and *in vivo.*[87] These patients also had decreases in PSA levels during the PC-SPES therapy.

PC-SPES has been found in multiple clinical trials to be an effective treatment for many patients with prostate cancer, even patients who did not respond to initial treatment with hormonal blockade.[88-90]

Further research will be necessary to ascertain which prostate cancer patients are most likely to benefit from PC-SPES treatment. There is no evidence to support the use of PC-SPES in cancers of organs other than the prostate.

Dosage and Toxicity:

Most patients in these studies were treated with three 320 mg capsules three times per day. Each of these clinical trials identified side effects of the treatment, including low libido, breast tenderness and increased propensity for blood clots.

SAW PALMETTO

Saw palmetto is one of the most commonly used herbal supplements in the world. It is commonly prescribed by herbal practitioners for the treatment of benign prostatic hyperplasia (BPH), a condition marked by enlargement of the prostate. Because of the shrinking effect that this herb has on the prostate, saw palmetto is sometimes suggested for cancers of this organ, as well. Saw palmetto is listed in some old herbal texts as a treatment for breast cancer.

Evidence:

Saw palmetto has been repeatedly found to prevent and treat benign prostatic hyperplasia. BPH, while not a malignant condition, is believed to share many common physiologic factors with prostate cancer in its development. A study of saw palmetto extract found that application of the extract to prostate cancer cells effectively inhibited the proliferation of these cells.[91] Several other *in vitro* studies have identified saw palmetto as a compound worthy of further study in the treatment of prostate cancer, as it has been found to induce apoptosis in prostate cancer cell lines.[92]

The safety of therapeutic doses of saw palmetto has been well-established in a number of clinical trials.[93] A double-blind, randomized controlled trial involving 27 patients aged 49 to 81 years with stage I or II prostate adenomas found that Saw palmetto extract improved urinary symptoms in 42.9% of patients compared to only 15.4% of those receiving placebo.[94] An additional study found that saw Saw palmetto blocked the conversion of testosterone to dihydrotestosterone *in vivo*.[95] This conversion is known to be one of the key mechanisms in the development and growth of prostate cancer. A different study found that Serenoa repens extract lowered testosterone levels in the blood.[96]

Saw palmetto is a component of the herbal cancer treatment PC-SPES discussed above, but it is not currently clear how much of the action of this formula can be attributed to any one herb.

Dosage and Toxicity:

Phase I clinical trials have established maximum tolerated dosages for saw palmetto, although its toxicity has not been fully studied. A typical and widely used dose is 320 mg of standardized herbal extract per day.

ESSIAC TEA

Rene Caisse, a Canadian nurse, first used the herbal mixture that bears her name (Essiac is Caisse spelled backwards) to treat patients with cancer in 1922. Her formula, which is reportedly based on a traditional Native American cancer treatment, contains four herbs: sheep sorrel, burdock, slippery elm and Indian rhubarb. Another commercially available version of Essiac contains watercress, kelp, blessed thistle and red clover, in addition to the herbs listed in the original formula.

The Essiac treatment generated controversy in Canada in the middle part of the last century. At one point, over 50,000 Canadians signed a petition to allow Ms. Caisse to continue to treat patients with her herbal compound.

A large number of anecdotal reports have testified to successful cancer treatment with the Essiac formula. The suggested benefits of Essiac included improved quality of life, pain relief and slowed progression of cancers.[97]

Evidence:

No published clinical trials have analyzed the effectiveness or safety of Essiac or other Essiac-like formulas. A multi-center clinical trial of the effectiveness of Essiac as a cancer treatment is in the planning stages at the National Cancer Institute of Canada, however.

Dosage and Toxicity:

Oral dosages of Essiac vary widely. This formula has been used as a tea, as whole-herb capsules and as an alcohol tincture. Essiac tends to be well tolerated, and no reports of serious toxicities have been reported.

Reports exist of intravenous use of Essiac. The safety of this procedure has not been established by clinical study.

HOXSEY FORMULA

The Hoxsey formula is an herbal mixture named after its first public proponent, Harry Hoxsey (1901–1974). His formula has been used to treat patients with cancer since at least 1919, and some reports suggest that other family members had also used it for nearly a century prior. The constituents of the original Hoxsey formula have been somewhat shrouded in secrecy. Dr. Hoxsey himself reported multiple versions of his formula. Regardless of the confusion, most versions of the Hoxsey formula reported in various sources contain similar components, including licorice root, red clover, poke root, burdock root, cascara sagrada, stillengia root, berberis root, prickly ash bark and potassium iodide.

Following several high profile battles with the American Medical Association in the mid-20th century, Hoxsey relocated his clinic to Mexico, where it remains to this day.

Evidence:

In vitro and animal research has shown a number of the constituents of the Hoxsey formula to have anticancer activity, including the ability to initiate cancer cell death and inhibit the promotion of existing tumors.[98-100] No studies of this type have analyzed the formula as a whole. While this treatment is thought to have few toxic effects when used as directed, several of the herbs in the Hoxsey formula could have severe side effects at higher doses.

Dr. Hoxsey reported the results of successfully treated cancer patients in a 1956 book entitled *"You Don't Have To Die."* Independent, controlled research has not confirmed the usefulness of the Hoxsey formula in the treatment of cancer.

At least two outside reviews of the Hoxsey clinic have been published. The first, from 1957, concluded that there was no evidence found upon chart review that internal use of the Hoxsey herbs had any effect on the progression of malignant disease.[101]

In the second report, 39 patients in the waiting room of the Hoxsey Clinic were asked to become part of a long-term follow-up study. While the majority of these patients either died or were otherwise lost to follow-up over the ensuing five years, six long-term survivors were identified.[102] At least two of these long-term survivors had advanced disease at the beginning of the study, and would not have been predicted to survive for five years with conventional treatment.

An unpublished case report of 9 patients with various types of cancer, written by authors at the Hoxsey clinic, found that the use of the Hoxsey formula had "positive benefits" in all cases.[103] All but one of these patients had prior conventional treatment.

Dosage and Toxicity:

Recommended dosages of this formula vary by source. Generally, 1-2 tsp of powdered herbs or alcohol tincture have been used two or three times per day. While this treatment is thought to have few toxic effects when used as directed, several of the herbs in the Hoxsey formula could have severe side effects at higher doses.

NONI

The juice of the fruit from a plant commonly known as noni (Morinda citrifolia) is marketed as a treatment for a number of conditions, including cancer. Noni is a plant found widely throughout the islands of the South Pacific. While noni is not found in any of the historical Western herbal medicine textbooks, anecdotal accounts of a historical use of noni as a cancer treatment exist.

Evidence:

In vitro and animal studies have shown promising effects of noni in multiple tumor models.[104-106] The researchers concluded that noni likely exerts its effect through enhancement of immune function. An additional study found that noni works to prevent cancer cell formation at the very early stages of the process.[107]

No human studies have assessed the efficacy of noni to treat patients with cancer or any other health condition.

Dosage and Toxicity:

Commonly used doses of noni juice (one ounce per day is a usual recommendation) are not reported to cause significant adverse reactions. Controlled research has not demonstrated the safety or efficacy of noni.

MGN-3

MGN-3 is a compound called an arabinoxylane isolated from rice bran. It is specially modified in a proprietary manner with enzymes from the Shiitake mushroom. Although MGN-3 uses mushrooms in its manufacture, it should not be confused with mushroom extracts such as PSK or PSP discussed above. But like these mushroom extracts, MGN-3 is thought to be an immune-stimulating treatment.

The company that makes MGN-3 was served an injunction in 1999 by the FDA for unlawful marketing of this product to patients with cancer and AIDS. The basis of the FDA action was that the product advertising made claims that were unsupported by scientific proof. The manufacturers of MGN-3 have denied any illegal marketing strategies.

Evidence:

There is some preliminary clinical research sponsored by the manufacturers showing that cancer patients with low immune function will have a dramatic increase in immune activity after treatment with MGN-3. No peer-reviewed research has confirmed this finding.

No published research has shown a direct benefit as far as tumor shrinkage or improved quality of life in cancer patients taking MGN-3. Anecdotal reports of anticancer benefits have been circulated by the manufacturers of MGN-3.

Dosage and Toxicity:

The usual dosage of MGN-3 for cancer patients is four capsules three times per day for a brief period, then two capsules twice daily thereafter. No serious adverse effects have been noted from this treatment. No peer-reviewed research has identified an optimal dose or demonstrated the long-term safety of this product.

1 Schink M. Mistletoe therapy for human cancer: the role of the natural killer cells. Anticancer Drugs 1997; 8:S47-51.

2 Khwaja TA, Dias CB, Pentecost S. Recent studies on the anticancer activities of mistletoe (Viscum album) and its alkaloids. Oncology 1986; 43:42-50.

3 Jung ML, Baudino S, Ribereau-Gayon G, et al. Characterization of cytotoxic proteins from mistletoe (Viscum album L.). Cancer Letters 1990; 51:103-8.

4 Janssen O, Scheffler A, Kabelitz D. In vitro effects of mistletoe extracts and mistletoe lectins. Arzneimittel-Forschung 1993; 43:1221-7.

5 Bradley GW, Clover A. Apparent response of small cell lung cancer to an extract of mistletoe. Thorax 1989; 44:1047-8.

6 Kuehn JJ. Favorable long-term outcome with mistletoe therapy in patients with centroblastic-centrocytic non Hodgkin's lymphoma. Deutsche Medizinische Wochenschrift 1999; 124:1414-8.

7 Salzer G, Havelec L. Prevention of recurrence of bronchial carcinomas after surgery by means of the mistletoe extract Iscador. Results of a clinical study from 1969-1971. Onkologie 1970, 1.264-7.

8 Grossarth-Maticek R, Kiene H, Baumgartner SM, et al. Use of Iscador, an extract of European mistletoe (Viscum album), in cancer treatment: prospective nonrandomized and randomized matched-pair studies nested within a cohort study. Alternative Therapies in Health and Medicine 2001; 7:57-66.

9 Lenartz D, Dott U, Menzel J, et al. Survival of glioma patients after complementary treatment with galactoside-specific lectin from mistletoe. Anticancer Research 2000; 20:2073-6.

10 Hajto T, et al. Increased secretion of tumor necrosis factor alpha, Interleukin 1, Interleukin 6 by human mononuclear cells exposed to b-Galatoside-specific Lectin from applied mistletoe extract. Cancer Research 1990; 50:3322-6.

11 Stumpf C, Bussing A. Stimulation of antitumour immunity by intrapleural instillation of a Viscum album L. extract. Anticancer Drugs 1997; 8 Suppl:S23-6.

12 Salzer G, et al. Does it make any sense to use mistletoe in the treatment of surgically incurable stomach cancer? Chirurgische Gastroentrologie Mit Interdisziplinaren Gesprachen 1989:2.

13 Salzer G. Pleura carcinosis. Cytomorphological findings with the mistletoe preparation iscador and other pharmaceuticals. Oncology 1986; 44:1047-8.

14 Boie D, Gutsch J, Burkhardt R. Treatment of liver metastases from various primary tumors with a Viscum preparation. Therapiewoche 1981; 31:1865-9.

15 Friess H, Beger HG, Kunz J, et al. Treatment of advanced pancreatic cancer with mistletoe: results of a pilot trial. Anticancer Research 1996; 16:915-20.

16 Kjaer M. Mistletoe (Iscador) therapy in stage IV renal adenocarcinoma. A phase II study in patients with measurable lung metastasis. Acta Oncologica 1989; 28:489-94.

17 McNamee D. Mistletoe extract ineffective in melanoma. Lancet 1999; 354:1101.

18 Stoss M, van Wely M, Musielsky H, et al. Study on local inflammatory reactions and other parameters during subcutaneous mistletoe application in HIV-positive patients and HIV-negative subjects over a period of 18 weeks. Arzneimittelforschung 1999; 49:366-73.

19 Kidd PM. The use of mushroom glucans and proteoglycans in cancer treatment. Alternative Medicine Review 2000; 5:4-27.

20 Tsukagoshi S, Hashimoto Y, Fujii G, et al. Krestin (PSK). Cancer Treatment Review 1984; 11:131-55.

21 Mao XW, Green LM, Gridley DS. Evaluation of polysaccharopeptide effects against C6 glioma in combination with radiation. Oncology 2001; 61:243-53.

22 Fujita H, Ogawa K, et al. Effect of PSK, a protein-bound polysaccharide from Coriolus versicolor on drug-metabolizing enzymes in sarcoma-180 bearing and normal mice. International Journal of Immunopharmacology 1988; 10:445-50.

23 Kobayashi H, Matsunaga K, Oguchi Y, Antimetastatic effects of PSK (Krestin), a protein-bound polysaccharide obtained from basidiomycetes: an overview. Cancer Epidemiology, Biomarkers and Prevention 1995; 4:275-81.

24 Yang MM, Chen Z, Kwok JS. The antitumor effect of a small polypeptide from Coriolus versicolor (SPCV). American Journal of Chinese Medicine 1992; 20:221-32.

25 Hsieh TC, Wu JM. Cell growth and gene modulatory activities of Yunzhi (Windsor Wunxi) from mushroom Trametes versicolor in androgen-dependent and androgen-insensitive human prostate cancer cells. International Journal of Oncology 2001; 18:81-8.

26 Hayakawa K, Mitsuhashi N, Saito Y, et al. Effect of Krestin (PSK) as adjuvant treatment on the prognosis after radical radiotherapy in patients with non-small cell lung cancer. Anticancer Research 1993; 13:1815-20.

27 Nakazato H, Koike A, Saji S, et al. Efficacy of immunochemotherapy as adjuvant treatment after curative resection of gastric cancer. Lancet 1994; 343:1122-6.

28 Torisu M, Hayashi Y, Ishimitsu T, et al. Significant prolongation of disease-free period gained by oral polysaccharide K (PSK) administration after curative surgical operation of colorectal cancer. Cancer Immunology, Immunotherapy 1990; 31:261-8.

29 Nagao T, Komatsuda M, Yamauchi K, et al. Chemoimmunotherapy with Krestin in acute leukemia. Tokai Journal of Experimental Clinical Medicine 1981; 6:141-6.

30 Kobayashi H, et al. Antimetastatic effects of PSK (Krestin), a protein-bound polysaccharide obtained from basidiomycetes: an overview. Cancer Epidemiology, Biomarkers & Prevention 1995; 4:275-81.

31 Ito H, et al. Antitumor effects of a new polysaccharide-protein complex (Atom) prepared from agaicus blazei (Iwade strain 101) himematsutake and its mechanisms in tumor-bearing mice. Anticancer Research 1997; 17:277-84.

32 Ogoshi K, Satou H, Isono K, Mitomi T, Endoh M, Sugita M. Possible predictive markers of immunotherapy in esophageal cancer.: Retrospective analysis of a randomized study. Cancer Investigation 1995; 13:363-9.

33 Ogoshi K, Satou H, Isono K, et al. Immunotherapy for esophageal cancer: A randomized trial in combination with radiotherapy and radiochemotherapy. American Journal of Clinical Oncology 1995; 18:216-22.

34 Nakazato H, et al. Efficacy of immunochemotherapy as adjuvant treatment after curative resection of gastric cancer. Lancet 1994; 343:1122-6.

35 Ohno R, et al. A randomized trial of chemoimmunotherapy of acute nonlymphocytic leukemia in adults using a protein-bound polysaccharide preparation. Cancer Immunology, Immunotherapy 1984; 18:149-54.

36 Iino Y, Yokoe T, Maemura M, et al. Immunochemotherapies versus chemotherapy as adjuvant treatment after curative resection of operable breast cancer. Anticancer Research 1995; 15:2907-15.

37 Fukushima S, Wanibuchi H, Li W. Inhibition by ginseng of colon carcinogenesis in rats. Journal of Korean Medical Science 2001; 16:S75-80.

38 Xiaoguang C, et al. Cancer chemopreventive and therapeutic activities of red ginseng. Journal of Ethnopharmacology 1998; 60:71-8.

39 Cha RJ, Zeng DW, Chang QS. Nonsurgical treatment of small cell lung cancer with chemo-radio-immunotherapy and traditional Chinese medicine. Zhonghua Nei Ke Za Zhi 1994; 33:462-6. [Chinese]

40 Tode T, Kikuchi Y, et al. In vitro and in vivo effects of ginsenoside Rh2 on the proliferation of serous cystadenocarcinoma of the human ovary. Nippon Sanka Fujinka Gakkai Zasshi 1992; 44:589-94.

41 Lee SJ, et al. Antitumor activity of a novel ginseng saponin metabolite in human pulmonary adenocarcinoma cells resistant to cisplatin. Cancer Letters 1999; 144:39-43.

42 Bohn B, Nebe CT, Birr C. Flow-cytometric studies with Eleutherococcus senticosus extract as an immunomodulatory agent. Arzneimittelforschung 1987; 37:1193-6.

43 Scaglione F, Ferrara F, Dugnani S, et al. Immunomodulatory effects of two extracts of Panax ginseng C.A. Meyer. Drugs Under Experimental and Clinical Research 1990; 16:537-42.

44 Srisurapanon S, Rungroeng K, Apibal S, et al. The effect of standardized ginseng extract on peripheral blood leukocyte subsets: a preliminary study in young healthy adults. Journal of the Medical Association of Thailand 1997; 80:S81-5.

45 Li NQ. Clinical and experimental study on shen-qi injection with chemotherapy in the treatment of malignant tumor of digestive tract. Zhongguo Zhong Xi Yi Jie He Za Zhi 1992; 12:588-92. [Chinese]

46 Cha RJ, Zeng DW, Chang QS. Non-surgical treatment of small cell lung cancer with chemo-radio-immunotherapy and traditional Chinese medicine. Zhonghua Nei Ke Za Zhi 1994; 33:462-6. [Chinese]

47 Kamei T, Kumano H, Iwata K, et al. The effect of a traditional Chinese prescription for a case of lung carcinoma. Journal of Alternative and Complementary Medicine 2000; 6:557-9.

48 Starosel'skii IV, Lisetskii VA, Kaban AP, et al. Prevention of postoperative complications in the surgical treatment of cancer of the lung, esophagus, stomach, large intestine and the rectum in patients over 60 years old. Voprosy Onkologii 1991; 37:873-7. [Russian]

49 Kupin VI, Polevaia EB. Stimulation of the immunological reactivity of cancer patients by Eleutherococcus extract. Voprosy Onkologii 1986; 32:21-6. [Russian]

50 Goel A, Boland CR, Chauhan DP. Specific inhibition of cyclooxygenase-2 (COX-2) expression by dietary curcumin in HT-29 human colon cancer cells. Cancer Letters 2001; 172:111-8.

51 Masferrer J. Approach to angiogenesis inhibition based on cyclooxygenase-2. Cancer Journal 2001; 7.3144-

52 Satoskar RR, Shah SJ, Shenoy SG. Evaluation of anti-inflammatory property of curcumin (diferuloyl methane) in patients with postoperative inflammation. International Journal of Clinical Pharmacology, Therapy and Toxicology 1986; 24:651-4.

53 Sreejayan N, Rao MNA. Free radical scavenging activity of curcuminoids. Arzneimittelforschung 1996; 46:169-71.

54 Ruby AJ, Kuttan G, Babu KD, et al. Antitumour and antioxidant activity of natural curcuminoids. Cancer Letters 1995; 94:79-83.

55 Bush JA, Cheung KJ Jr, Li G. Curcumin induces apoptosis in human melanoma cells through Fas receptor/caspase-8 pathway independent of p53. Experimental Cell Research 2001; 271:305-14.

56 Jee SH, Shen SC, Tseng CR, Chiu HC, Kuo ML. Curcumin induces a p53-dependent apoptosis in human basal carcinoma cells. Journal of Investigative Dermatology 1998; 111:656-61.

57 Dorai T, et al. Therapeutic potential of curcumin in human prostate cancer. Curcumin inhibits proliferation, induces apoptosis, and inhibits angiogenesis of LNCaP prostate cancer cells in vivo. Prostate 2001; 47:293-303.

58 Chuang SE, et al. Curcumin-containing diet inhibits diethylnitrosamine-induced murine hepatocarcinogenesis. Carcinogenesis 2000; 21:331-5.

59 Cheng AL, Hsu CH, Lin JK, et al. Phase I clinical trial of curcumin, a chemopreventive agent, in patients with high-risk or pre-malignant lesions. Anticancer Research 2001; 21:2895-900.

60 Sharma RA, McLelland HR, Hill KA, et al. Pharmacodynamic and pharmacokinetic study of oral Curcuma extract in patients with colorectal cancer. Clinical Cancer Research 2001; 7:1894-900.

61 Cheng AL, Hsu CH, Lin JK, et al. Phase I clinical trial of curcumin, a chemopreventive agent, in patients with high-risk or pre-malignant lesions. Anticancer Research 2001; 21:2895-900.

62 Sharma RA, McLelland HR, Hill KA, et al. Pharmacodynamic and pharmacokinetic study of oral Curcuma extract in patients with colorectal cancer. Clinical Cancer Research 2001; 7:1894-900.

63 Zhao KS, Mancini C, Doria G. Enhancement of the immune response in mice by Astragalus membranaceus extracts. Immunopharmacology 1990; 20:225-33.

64 Qun L, Luo Q, Zhang ZY, et al. Effects of astragalus on IL-2/IL-2R system in patients with maintained hemodialysis. Clinical Nephrology 1999; 52:333-4.

65 Zhao KW, Kong HY. Effect of Astragalan on secretion of tumor necrosis factors in human peripheral blood mononuclear cells. Zhongguo Zhong Xi Yi Jie He Za Zhi 1993; 13:263-5, 259.

66 Chu DT, Lin JR, Wong W. The in vitro potentiation of LAK cell cytotoxicity in cancer and aids patients induced by F3—a fractionated extract of Astragalus membranaceus. Zhonghua Zhong Liu Za Zhi 1994; 16:167-71.

67 Chu D, et al. F3, a fractionated extract of Astragalus membranaceus, potentiates lymphokine-activated killer cell cytotoxicity generated by low-dose recombinant interleukin-2. Zhongguo Zhong Xi Yi Jie He Za Zhi 1990; 10:34-6.

[68] Li NQ. Clinical and experimental study on shen-qi injection with chemotherapy in the treatment of malignant tumor of digestive tract. Zhongguo Zhong Xi Yi Jie He Za Zhi 1992; 12:588-92. [Chinese]

[69] Zhang XQ, Liu SJ, Pan XY. Clinical study on treatment of chemo- or radiotherapy induced leukopenia with fuzheng compound. Zhongguo Zhong Xi Yi Jie He Za Zhi 1996; 16:27-8. [Chinese]

[70] Kamei T, Kumano H, Iwata K, Nariai Y, Matsumoto T. The effect of a traditional Chinese prescription for a case of lung carcinoma. Journal of Alternative and Complementary Medicine 2000 Dec; 6:557-9.

[71] Piscoya J, Rodriguez Z, Bustamante SA, et al. Efficacy and safety of freeze-dried cat's claw in osteoarthritis of the knee: mechanisms of action of the species Uncaria guianensis. Inflammation Research 2001; 50:442-8

[72] Sheng Y, Bryngelsson C, Pero RW. Enhanced DNA repair, immune function and reduced toxicity of C-MED-100, a novel aqueous extract from Uncaria tomentosa. Journal of Ethnopharmacology 2000; 69:115-26.

[73] Riva L, Coradini D, Di Fronzo G, et al. The antiproliferative effects of Uncaria tomentosa extracts and fractions on the growth of breast cancer cell line. Anticancer Research 2001; 21:2457-61.

[74] Oswald H. Case reports (unpublished).

[75] Immodal Pharmaka; Therapy records over a 10-year-period. Krallendorn-Medicaments: Special Information for Physicians and Dispensing Chemists. 2nd Revised ed. Austria: 1993; 16-7.

[76] Piscoya J, Rodriguez Z, Bustamante SA, et al. Efficacy and safety of freeze-dried cat's claw in osteoarthritis of the knee: mechanisms of action of the species Uncaria guianensis. Inflammation Research 2001; 50:442-8.

[77] Pienta KJ, Naik H, Akhtar A, et al. Inhibition of spontaneous metastasis in a rat prostate cancer model by oral administration of modified citrus pectin. Journal of the National Cancer Institute 1995; 87:348-53.

[78] Platt D, Raz A. Modulation of the lung colonization of B16-F1 melanoma cells by citrus pectin. Journal of the National Cancer Institute 1992; 84:438-42.

[79] Hayashi A, Gillen AC, Lott JR. Effects of daily oral administration of quercetin chalcone and modified citrus pectin. Alternative Medicine Review 2000; 5:546-52.

[80] Avivi-Green C, Polak-Charcon S, Madar Z, Schwartz B. Apoptosis cascade proteins are regulated in vivo by high intracolonic butyrate concentration:correlation with colon cancer inhibition. Oncology Research 2000; 12:83-95.

[81] Hsieh TC, Wu JM. Changes in cell growth, cyclin/kinase, endogenous phosphoproteins and nm23 gene expression in human prostatic JCA-1 cells treated with modified citrus pectin. Biochemistry and Molecular Biology International 1995; 37:833-41.

[82] Strum S, Scholz M, McDermed J, et al. Modified citrus pectin slows PSA doubling time: a pilot clinical trial. Presentation: International Conference on Diet and Prevention of Cancer, Tampere, Finland. 1999.

[83] Ikezoe T, Chen SS, Heber D, Taguchi H, Koeffler HP. Baicalin is a major component of PC-SPES which inhibits the proliferation of human cancer cells via apoptosis and cell cycle arrest. Prostate 2001; 49:292-5.

[84] Kubota T, et al. PC-SPES: a unique inhibitor of proliferation of prostate cancer cells in vitro and in vivo. Prostate 2000; 42:163-71.

[85] Oh WK, George DJ, Kantoff PW. Rapid rise of serum prostate specific antigen levels after discontinuation of the herbal therapy PC-SPES in patients with advanced prostate carcinoma: report of four cases. Cancer 2002; 94:686-9.

[86] de la Taille A, et al. Role of herbal compounds (PC-SPES) in hormone-refractory prostate cancer: two case reports. Journal of Alternative and Complementary Medicine 2000; 6:449-51.

[87] de la Taille A, et al. Herbal therapy PC-SPES: in vitro effects and evaluation of its efficacy in 69 patients with prostate cancer. Journal of Urology 2000; 164:1229-34.

[88] Small EJ, Frohlich MW, Bok R, et al. Prospective trial of the herbal supplement PC-SPES in patients with progressive prostate cancer. Journal of Clinical Oncology 2000; 18:3595-603.

[89] De La Taille A, Buttyan R, Hayek O, et al. Herbal therapy PC-SPES: in vitro effects and evaluation of its efficacy in 69 patients with prostate cancer. Journal of Urology 2000; 164:1229-34.

90 DiPaola RS, Zhang H, Lambert GH, et al. Clinical and biologic activity of an estrogenic herbal combination (PC-SPES) in prostate cancer. New England Journal of Medicine 1998; 339:785-91.

91 Ishii K, et al. Extract from Serenoa repens suppresses the invasion activity of human urological cancer cells by inhibiting urokinase-type plasminogen activator. Biolgical and Pharmacological Bulletin 2001; 24:188-190.

92 Iguchi K, Okumura N, Usui S, et al. Myristoleic acid, a cytotoxic component in the extract from Serenoa repens, induces apoptosis and necrosis in human prostatic LNCaP cells. Prostate 2001; 47:59-65.

93 Boyle P, Robertson C, Lowe F, et al. Meta-analysis of clinical trials of permixon in the treatment of symptomatic benign prostatic hyperplasia. Urology 2000; 55:533-9.

94 Di Silverio F, et al. Evidence that Serenoa repens extract displays an antiestrogenic activity in prostatic hypertrophy patients. European Urology 1992; 21:309-314.

95 Boik J. Cancer and Natural Medicine: A Textbook of Basic Science and Clinical Research; Oregon Medical Press. Princeton, Minn, 1995.

96 Pannunzio E, et al. Serenoa repens in the treatment of human benign prostatic hypertrophy (BPH). Journal of Urology 1987; 137.

97 Tamayo C, Richardson MA, Diamond S, Skoda L. The chemistry and biological activity of herbs used in Flor-Essence herbal tonic and Essiac. Phytotherapy Research 2000; 14:1-14.

98 Zhang RX, Dougherty DV, Rosenblum ML. Laboratory studies of berberine used alone and in combination with 1,3-bis (2-chloroethyl)-1-nitrosourea to treat malignant brain tumors. Chinese Medical Journal (English) 1990; 103:658-65.

99 Ju Y, Still CC, Sacalis JN, et al. Cytotoxic coumarins and lignans from extracts of the northern prickly ash (Zanthoxylum americanum). Phytotherapy Research 2001; 15:441-3.

100 Wang HB, Zheng QY. Effects of Phytolacca acinosa polysaccharides I with different schedules on its antitumor efficiency in tumor bearing mice and production of IL-1, IL-2, IL-6, TNF, CSF activity in normal mice. Immunopharmacology and Immunotoxicology 1997; 19:197-213.

101 Mather JM, Carrethers AWR, Harlow N, et al. Report of a committee of faculty members of the University of British Columbia concerning the Hoxsey Treatment for cancer. Vancouver: University of British Columbia, 1957.

102 Austin S, Dale EB, DeKadt S. Long term follow-up of cancer patients using Contreras, Hoxsey, and Gerson therapies. Journal of Naturopathic Medicine 1995; 5:75-6.

103 Biomedical Center (Hoxsey clinic). Information on the hoxsey therapy. (Tijuana, Mexico).

104 Hirazumi A, Furusawa E. An immunomodulatory polysaccharide-rich substance from the fruit juice of Morinda citrifolia (noni) with antitumour activity. Phytotherapy Research 1999; 13:380-7.

105 Hirazumi A, Furusawa E, Chou SC, et al. Immunomodulation contributes to the anti-cancer activity of Morinda citrifolia (noni) fruit juice. Proceedings of the Western Pharmacology Society 1996; 39:7-9.

106 Hiramatsu T, Imoto M, Koyano T, et al. Induction of normal phenotypes in ras-transformed cells by damnacanthal from Morinda citrifolia. Cancer Letters 1993; 73:161 6.

107 Wang MY, Su C. Cancer Preventive of Morinda citrifolia (Noni). Annals of the New York Academy of Medicine 2001; 952:161-8.

Chapter Six

Diet-Related Therapies and Regimens

This chapter details various approaches that include nutrition or a particular supplement as part of an overall anti-cancer therapy. These systems are usually practiced in a clinic where randomized clinical research is not being conducted. A total program of lifestyle change may produce psychological benefits in adherents to a particular regimen that are unrelated to whether that regimen is affecting tumor biology. Many cancer survivors cannot afford to take part in these clinics and so construct their own lifestyle programs by borrowing from many different dietary and lifestyle philosophies.

Can any of these systems work as well as, or better than, traditional anticancer therapies? The National Center for Complementary and Alternative Medicine (NCCAM) is beginning to investigate these approaches and is funding the study of Complementary and Alternative Medicine (CAM) therapies in a number of cancer centers nationally.

This chapter includes several diet-related therapies and approaches that are based on theories currently at odds with conventional knowledge and published literature. In all cases, the most up-to-date information on these regimens and therapies available is provided so that you and your doctor can discuss these approaches intelligently.

MELATONIN

Melatonin is a hormone secreted from a gland in the brain called the pineal gland. This hormone is secreted in largest quantities at night, and is thought to be part of the body's way of signaling its requirement for sleep. Melatonin is available over the counter and is often used at low doses as a natural sleep aid.

Evidence:

Recent studies suggest that melatonin may have effects on the immune system and on cell-to-cell signaling. Melatonin is believed by some researchers to be part of a class of molecules known as biological response modifiers, which are agents that either change immune function or regulate the way in which cancer cells divide.

Melatonin has several potential mechanisms of action that may be partially responsible for its reported anti-cancer effects. It is a potent antioxidant, and may protect against free radical damage to the genes. Melatonin reduces secretion of a compound called tumor necrosis factor,[1] a signaling molecule that may be responsible for weight loss, low blood counts and poor appetite seen in advanced cancer patients.

In *in vitro* studies, melatonin blocks secretion of prostaglandins, which are cell messengers that promote tumor cell growth. It is not known currently which, if any, of these mechanisms are most important to the effect of melatonin treatment seen in the studies discussed below. Melatonin is also known to stimulate apoptosis, or cell death, in cancer cells.[2]

Recently, studies have begun to investigate the use of melatonin in groups of cancer patients. It should be noted that, to date, most of these clinical studies involving melatonin have been conducted by the same group of authors, and were not placebo-controlled.

Melatonin has been reported to inhibit the proliferation of human prostate cancer cells transplanted into mice.[3] Researchers have also reported that melatonin can improve cancer chemotherapy. In this study, researchers discovered that melatonin enhanced the therapeutic ability of diamminedichloroplatinum to kill ovarian cancer cells.[4]

As a sole agent, melatonin has been reported to lead to a stabilization of disease in up to 40% of advanced cancer patients, together with an increased sense of well-being.[1] In patients with metastases to the brain from solid tumors, addition of melatonin to standard supportive care significantly improved average survival times, while reducing complications from steroid treatment.[5] Melatonin treatment has also been shown to be more effective than supportive care alone for maintaining weight in late stage cancer.[6] In a group of patients receiving chemotherapy for advanced solid tumors (including lung, breast and gastrointestinal cancers), patients taking melatonin were over twice as likely to survive for one year as those only receiving chemotherapy treatment.[7] Another study found similar improvement in survival statistics in lung cancer patients taking melatonin compared to those only on chemotherapy.[8] In a small study of patients with highly malignant brain tumors, addition of melatonin to radiation therapy improved one-year survival (from 7% to 43%) compared to radiation alone.[9]

A study of 20 metastatic cancer patients found that 20 mg per day of melatonin administered in the evening for 2 months produced minor response in 2 patients, stable disease in 6 others, and progressive disease in the remaining 12 patients.[10] The researchers found that melatonin reduced the levels of vascular endothelial growth factor (VEGF) in the serum of these patients. VEGF has been found to be an important factor in the growth of cancer because it increases the blood supply to growing cancer tissues.

A Phase II study of 12 patients with several cancer types, including Hodgkin's disease, multiple myeloma, acute myelogenous leukemia, chronic myelomonocytic leukemia, and non-Hodgkin's lymphoma, found that 20 mg per day of melatonin, given in the evening, led to the partial response of 1 patient, stable disease in 7 other patients, and disease progression in the other 4 patients.[11]

Dosage and Toxicity:

Most of the clinical trials using melatonin as a cancer treatment used a 20 mg dose. Doses as high as 40 mg have been studied, with no evidence of serious toxicity. Doses far in excess of this have been used in animal studies, again with no evidence of organ toxicity.

The most common adverse effects reported clinically with melatonin at the higher doses are fatigue, disturbed sleep and lucid dreaming. These effects are usually mild and reversible upon discontinuing treatment.

ANTINEOPLASTONS

Antineoplastons are a group of naturally occurring amino acid derivatives. Research began on these compounds in 1967, after a physician named Stanislaw Burzynski reported significant differences in the urinary amino acid content of cancer patients compared to healthy control subjects. Soon after, Dr. Burzynski reported that several of the antineoplastons had significant anticancer activity, combined with low toxicity.[12]

In 1995, Dr. Burzynski was indicted by a federal grand jury for mail fraud and marketing an unapproved drug. He was not convicted of these charges.

Dr. Burzynski has obtained consent to continue giving his treatment, but only under the auspices of clinical trials. He has yet to publish the results of any of these studies.

Evidence:

A number of published animal and *in vitro* studies have shown potential anti-cancer activity for the antineoplastons. Specifically, injection of antineoplastons has inhibited the growth of breast cancer and liver cancer cells transplanted into mice.[13,14] Antineoplastons have also induced the death of liver cancer cells in the lab.[15] Researchers have found that the levels of the antineoplaston A10 in the urine of breast cancer patients are negatively correlated with high apoptosis, or cell death, levels.[16] These researchers also found that antineoplaston A10 significantly inhibited neutrophil apoptosis *in vitro*.

A study has found that a deficiency of antineoplastons may be required for malignant cells to proliferate in the body.[17] A clinical trial published by the Mayo Clinic in 1999 examined the safety and efficacy of 2 antineoplastons (A10 and AS2-1) in patients with advanced brain tumors. In 6 patients with assessable outcomes (9 patients total were treated), no clinical responses were noted.[18] Significant neurotoxicity (confusion, elevation of sodium in the blood, vomiting, exacerbation of preexisting seizure disorders) was seen in 5 patients treated with the experimental compound.

Two reports by a group of researchers from a Japanese university suggest a clinical benefit from antineoplaston therapy used in combination with conventional therapies against several different types of cancer, including those of the lung and brain.[19,20] Controlled studies have yet to assess this combination approach.

A study of 20 patients with advanced brain cancer reported that A10 and AS infusions led to a complete or partial response in 6 patients. An additional 10 patients had stabilization of disease during the trial. A clinical series involving 25 patients with various types of stage III-V disease found that injections of A3 at 100 mg/ml led to a complete response in 5 patients, partial response in 5 others, and stable disease in 9 others.[21] The patients were started at 100 mg/ml of A3, and the dose was increased in 100 mg increments every 12 hours in most patients.

Another clinical series involving 19 bladder cancer patients without evidence of metastasis found that the use of A2, A3, A5, A10, or AS2-1 led to a complete response in 68% of patients and a relative response in 11%.[22] A different clinical series that included 42 patients with various types of advanced cancer found that 500 mg of A10 given in various doses and durations led to a positive response in 75% of cases.[23]

It should be noted that each of the positive results outlined above were published by Dr. Burzynski or members of his team, and have not yet been confirmed by independent investigators.

Dosage and Toxicity:

The antineoplaston treatment has become popular largely because of its comparative lack of side effects. The neurotoxicity seen in the Mayo Clinic study discussed above was the first report of serious adverse effects with this treatment.

CARTILAGE (Shark/Bovine)

Cartilage from cows and sharks has been studied for anticancer potential. Although several mechanisms have been theorized to explain cartilage's possible antitumor activity, the theory that is currently attracting the most scientific attention is that cartilage contains a protein or proteins that inhibit the formation of new blood vessels to supply tumors. The formation of these new blood vessels (called angiogenesis) is considered necessary for cancers to grow.

After a *60 Minutes* report highlighting the use of shark cartilage in Cuban cancer patients, this treatment gained much notoriety in the United States. Several commercial preparations of shark and bovine cartilage are currently available.

Evidence:

A few studies have investigated the possibility that bovine and shark cartilage may exert direct toxic effects on certain cancer cells *in vitro*, but a precise and plausible biological mechanism to explain how this may occur has not yet been offered. In one such study, high concentrations of bovine cartilage (1-5 mg/ml) were found to inhibit the growth of tumors of different origin and in three human cell lines (myeloma, breast cancer and colon cancer).[24] This study did not investigate the effects of bovine cartilage on healthy cells.

Another *in vitro* study found that a standard concentration (.75 mg/ml) of powdered shark cartilage had no effect upon the growth of astrocytoma cells (cancer arising from brain/spinal tissue.)[25]

Several laboratory studies have investigated the theory that bovine and shark cartilage may inhibit angiogenesis of cancer cells. Proteins in bovine cartilage have shown the ability to inhibit *in vitro* cell proliferation and blood vessel formation in chicken embryos, but have not been shown to block the *in vitro* proliferation of tumor cells.[26]

Shark cartilage has been estimated to contain 1,000 times more antiangiogenic potential than bovine cartilage.[27] Substances in shark cartilage have displayed a wide range of antiangiogenic activity *in vitro*, but have not been shown to inhibit the proliferation of cancer cells.[28]

In animal studies, shark cartilage has shown the ability to inhibit chemically-induced angiogenesis and reduce the growth of brain cancers in rats.[29,30] Shark cartilage was found to have no effect on skin cancer in mice.[31]

Three human studies on cartilage have been published to date. Two of these studies deal with bovine cartilage.

The first study was not a clinical study, but a case series of 31 advanced or recurrent cancer patients, most of whom received conventional cancer therapy before or during the period of the study. Bovine cartilage was administered in a variety of ways (orally, via injection or by topical application) depending on the patients' type of cancer. Dosage and duration of treatment varied widely, and there was no control group. Nineteen subjects experienced complete remission, 10 had a partial response, 1 patient had stable disease, 1 patient did not respond to treatment. Half of the patients with complete remission eventually developed recurrent cancer.[32]

A different clinical series involving 22 patients with renal cancer that had metastasized reported that a formulation of shark cartilage that contained 3 grams per day for 30 days led to complete response in 3 patients and that more than half had some shrinkage of lesions in the lungs.[33] A series of best-case reports that included 21 patients with late-stage cancers of various types found that shark cartilage use led to a reduction in tumor size in 61% of patients.[34] Overall, 87% of this group was found to have an improved quality of life.

A Phase II trial with bovine cartilage was undertaken with 9 patients, all of whom had progressive diseases following conventional therapy. Dosages (via injection) were standardized but duration of treatment varied widely due to disease progression and/or death. One patient with metastatic kidney cancer had a complete response for a period of 10 months. The other 8 patients did not respond to treatment. No significant effect on subjects' immune systems was apparent.[35]

The only published clinical trial of oral shark cartilage conducted to date involved 60 patients with various types of advanced solid tumors, 59 of whom had been previously treated by conventional means. None of the subjects in this study showed any clinical response to treatment.[36]

Currently, several clinical trials are underway. One trial will compare lung cancer patients taking shark cartilage with conventional therapy to subjects receiving only conventional therapy. Another trial will compare kidney cancer patients receiving shark cartilage to kidney cancer patients receiving a placebo. A Canadian study will investigate use of shark cartilage in patients with relapsed or refractory multiple myeloma.[37 39]

Shark cartilage will also be studied in a randomized Phase III clinical trial in patients with advanced breast or colorectal cancer.[40] Thus, the efficacy of this treatment is still unknown.

Dosage and Toxicity:

The optimal dose of cartilage has not been established. The only clinical trial using a standardized dose involved shark cartilage at a concentration of 1 g/kg of body weight (roughly 65 grams in an average adult). In this study, the adverse effects were generally mild and were mainly gastrointestinal in nature.

GERSON TREATMENT

Dr. Max Gerson (1881-1959) was an early proponent of the concept that diet has an influence on disease incidence in humans. His interest in diet began when he used dietary changes to treat his own migraine headaches. He gained prominence in Germany in the late 1920s, after successfully treating a number of patients with tuberculosis with dietary treatments. He began treating cancer patients with his dietary regimen around this time, as well.

After reviews of his patient outcomes by the National Cancer Institute and the New York County Medical Society, his therapies were widely critiqued – some would say discredited – in the scientific press. His therapy is still available at specialty clinics in Mexico and Arizona, and is practiced by several other physicians across the United States.

His therapy consists of many different interventions. These include a very low-salt diet, high intake of fresh fruit and vegetable juices, frequent coffee enemas, liver extract injections, high-dose thyroid medication and other therapies.

Dr. Gerson believed that his therapies worked by inducing detoxification of the body. Other explanations for this treatment strategy include manipulation of acid/base balance and stimulation of immune function. These theories have not been confirmed by independent research.

Evidence:

Dr. Gerson published a book entitled *A Cancer Therapy: Results of Fifty Cases* in 1958. In this book, he reported many cases of patients who he believed did much better than their prognosis would indicate. These reports were subsequently criticized on a number of grounds, including lack of pathological evidence in support of a cancer diagnosis and use of established therapies in addition.

More recently, a retrospective chart review study published by the Gerson Research Organization compared survival statistics for patients treated by the Gerson method to those treated by conventional medicine. They reported superior survival outcomes in all stages of melanoma (I-IV) with the Gerson treatment.[41] In a study by independent investigators, 21 patients at the Gerson Clinic were followed for 5 years or until death. Only 1 of these patients was still alive at the end of the five-year study.[42]

Dosage and Toxicity:

The Gerson diet is a very low-protein and low-sodium diet. The safety of such dramatic dietary changes in patients with cancer has not been established.

Coffee enemas can lead to serious complications in patients with compromised immunity, such as intestinal perforation and serious infections, and deaths have been reported from this procedure.[43,44] The doses of thyroid hormone used in the Gerson therapy are much higher than the daily output of a normal gland, and could also be associated with significant adverse effects.

MACROBIOTIC DIET

Macrobiotics is a diet and lifestyle treatment program based on principles drawn from Traditional Chinese Medicine. The leading modern proponent of this type of treatment is Michio Kushi. His Kushi Institute in Boston has published a number of works describing macrobiotic principles.

The macrobiotic diet contains very high amounts of whole grains, vegetables and legumes. It largely eschews red meat and dairy, and contains very small amounts of fish and poultry. Macrobiotic lifestyle recommendations describe proper chewing, bathing and clothing, among other things.

Evidence:

Michio Kushi has published a number of reports of cancer patients he believes have been successfully treated with his macrobiotic regimen. The theoretical benefits of macrobiotic diets have been described in detail elsewhere.[45] No controlled trials have measured the effect of this treatment program.

Dosage and Toxicity:

The safety of the macrobiotic diet has not been established in cancer patients. There are serious concerns about the macrobiotic diet in patients with cancer-related wasting, as this diet is very low in calories and protein. A macrobiotic diet can also lead to serious nutrient deficiencies in some individuals, as it lacks calcium, iron, riboflavin, vitamin B12 and other nutrients.[46]

LIVINGSTON METHOD

The Livingston method is named after Virginia Livingston, MD. She developed her treatment regimen in response to her belief that cancer was caused by infection with a bacterium she called progenitor cryptocides. Her belief was that the greatest chance for cure would come from improving immune function against this bacterial infection.

Her treatment protocol is complex and includes vaccine therapy (reportedly including vaccines made from patient urine), vegetarian diets, nutritional supplements, digestive enzymes, enemas and psychologic techniques. This treatment is still available through the Livingston-Wheeler Clinic.

Evidence:

Potential benefits of several of the components of her therapy, including dietary changes,[47] proteolytic enzymes[48] and nutritional supplements,[49] have some support in theory or in preliminary studies.

One study by independent investigators compared 78 advanced cancer patients under care at the Livingston-Wheeler Clinic with 78 patients receiving conventional treatment at a teaching hospital. Each had terminal disease with a predicted survival time of less than one year. Both groups of patients had average survival times of 15 months.[50] Quality of life scores tended to be better in patients treated with conventional medicine.

Dosage and Toxicity:

This treatment appears to be well tolerated according to Dr. Livingston. Patients undergoing this treatment should take special care to ensure that nutrient intake is adequate on the restricted diet. The safety of Dr. Livingston's vaccine treatment has not been demonstrated in clinical trials.

LAETRILE

Laetrile is a cyanide containing chemical compound derived from apricot pits that represents the most popular alternative cancer treatment of the last half century. Laetrile is sometimes referred to as amygdalin, although actually these are slightly different compounds. Some resources also refer to laetrile as vitamin B17, although it does not to meet the criteria for vitamin status (that is, it is not known to be necessary for normal human physiology).

Ernst Krebs, Sr., MD, with his son Ernst, Jr., began using laetrile in the 1950s. Laetrile gained some high-profile benefactors in the 1960s, and hence gained wide popularity at that time. Legal battles ensued, with the result that laetrile production and use was banned in the United States as toxic and ineffective. Several clinics presently provide laetrile treatment in Mexico.

Laetrile treatment is generally part of a more comprehensive treatment regimen. Diet changes, nutritional supplementation, and proteolytic enzymes are common adjuncts to laetrile therapy.

Laetrile is thought by proponents to be directly toxic to tumor cells, while being relatively non-toxic to healthy tissue. It is claimed that the action of laetrile is due to selective release of cyanide compounds in the tumors, taking advantage of metabolic differences between normal tissue and cancers.

Evidence:

In published reports of animal studies sponsored by the National Cancer Institute, laetrile had no effect against several different tumor types, including those of the breast, liver, lymph and blood (leukemic.)[51] There have been reports in the popular press of animal studies that showed a clear anti-cancer effect of laetrile, but these were never published in the scientific literature.

A preliminary, multi-center clinical trial with laetrile therapy was published in 1982. Of 178 late-stage cancer patients treated, researchers noted no evidence of disease response or cure.[52] Again, advocates of laetrile therapy have heavily critiqued this study.

Promising case reports of laetrile treatment have been published both in the scientific literature[53] and in the lay press. However, these reports have been criticized on several grounds, including poor proof of cancer diagnosis and concurrent use of standard therapies.

Dosage and Toxicity:

The optimal dose of laetrile for cancer therapy has been variously reported by different sources. Most sources suggest oral doses of between 1g and 10g of laetrile per day.

In the 1982 clinical trial, serious side effects were noted. These were thought to be due to excessive blood concentrations of cyanide.[52]

GONZALEZ/KELLEY METHOD

A cancer treatment regimen referred to either as the Gonzalez or the Kelley method is based on the work of a Scottish doctor named John Beard. Dr. Beard postulated in 1911 that cancer occurs due to a deficiency of proteolytic enzymes (enzymes that digest proteins), which in turn allows cancer to invade normal tissue. Supplementation with high doses of proteolytic enzymes from the cow pancreas is a major component of this treatment.

Dr. Kelley, a dentist from Texas, has been using his treatment protocol for many years. In addition to the enzymes discussed above, he advocates nutritional supplementation, a strict diet (ranging from vegetarian to mainly meat, depending on the situation), enemas, prayer and osteopathic-like manipulation.

Dr. Gonzalez learned about Kelley's treatment firsthand, and his treatment program varies only slightly. Like that of Dr. Kelley, the central tenets of his protocol are enzymes, diet changes and nutritional supplementation.

Both Dr. Kelley and Dr. Gonzalez use non-standard testing to monitor the progress of the disease. Dr. Kelley uses a questionnaire to classify patients by metabolic type. Dr. Gonzalez uses a hair test, reportedly based on an energetic diagnostic method called radionics that is not accepted in the medical literature.

Evidence:

In vitro, animal and human research has proposed many potential benefits of proteolytic enzyme therapy for patients with cancer.[54] Many of these benefits involve potentiation of conventional therapeutic agents while reducing the adverse effects of radiotherapy and chemotherapy. The potential benefits of the detoxification regimen and related changes, however, remain unproven and theoretical.

Dr. Gonzalez published a case series of 11 consecutive patients from his practice treated for pancreatic cancer. This paper, published in a peer-reviewed journal, concluded that 1-year survival in his patient population vastly exceeded that predicted from conventional treatment (81% v. 25%).[55] These results are reportedly being followed up with more formal clinical trials.

Dr. Kelley has never published results of his treatment in a peer-reviewed scientific journal.

The validity of the hair analysis used by Dr. Gonzalez or the diagnostic questionnaire used by Dr. Kelley have not been confirmed by other investigators.

Dosage and Toxicity:

Both of these treatment programs require very high dose nutritional and enzyme supplementation. A typical treatment protocol may require upwards of 100 pills to be taken each day.

Enemas can lead to serious, even fatal, infections in cancer patients with compromised immunity.[43,44]

HYDRAZINE SULFATE

Hydrazine sulfate is a simple chemical compound that has been touted as a treatment for late-stage cancer patients. Joseph Gold, MD, first proposed hydrazine sulfate as a treatment for the symptoms of muscle wasting and weight loss seen in advanced cancer patients. Early animal studies also suggested a direct anti-tumor effect of hydrazine sulfate.

Hydrazine sulfate therapy is widely used in Europe, particularly in Russia. In the United States, hydrazine sulfate is available to physicians through the Investigational New Drug program of the FDA. Proponents of this therapy believe that it can be used in any type of cancer and can be used concurrently with standard therapeutics.

Evidence:

The preliminary research with hydrazine sulfate suggested that it could potentially reverse some, but not all, of the metabolic changes that occur in late stage cancers.[56] These metabolic changes are responsible for a process called cachexia, which consists of weight loss and wasting.

Although a minority of studies suggested some inhibition of tumor growth with hydrazine sulfate therapy, the mechanism by which this may occur remains obscure.

The first clinical trials with hydrazine sulfate suggested that it was an effective prophylaxis against weight loss in advanced cancer patients.[57,58] The latter study also appeared to show a trend toward improved survival when hydrazine sulfate was added to chemotherapy for lung cancer.

Later trials performed at the Mayo Clinic failed to show any measurable benefit in terms of weight maintenance or survival time attributable to hydrazine sulfate.[59,60]

Perhaps due to less rigorous study design, studies from Russia have shown much higher incidence of tumor regression in patients treated with hydrazine sulfate.[61,62]

Dosage and Toxicity:

The usual dosage regimen for oral hydrazine sulfate is 60 mg 3 times daily for 30-45 days, followed by a 2-4 week rest period. This cycle is then repeated. Hydrazine sulfate is also available for injection.

There are generally few side effects from hydrazine sulfate when used as recommended.[57] Nausea, itching, dizziness, drowsiness and nerve damage have been reported.[56] Dr. Gold also recommends that hydrazine sulfate not be taken with alcohol and certain classes of tranquilizers.

There has been one published report of a fatal case of liver and renal failure associated with the use of hydrazine sulfate.[63] This effect has not been seen in clinical trials or in animal studies with this medication.

HOMEOPATHY

Homeopathy is a medical system founded in eighteenth century Germany by Dr. Samuel Hahnemann. Homeopathic physicians believe in the use of extremely dilute medicines, often from a natural source. Many homeopathic medicines are in fact so dilute that they are not likely to contain a single molecule of the original substance. Advocates of homeopathy maintain that these dilute medicines retain the healing energy of the original substance without the potential for toxicity.

Evidence:

Whether or not the dilute remedies of homeopathy have a physiological effect has been a matter of intense debate in the medical community for over two hundred years. There is no published research showing a plausible mechanism for the benefits that doctors of homeopathy have reported for cancer patients. Most advocates of homeopathy believe that modern science lacks the ability to measure the action of homeopathic medicines at a molecular level.

No modern clinical studies have assessed the anti-cancer effect of homeopathic medicine. The evidence in favor of homeopathy in the treatment of cancer is currently anecdotal. Homeopathic doctors have reported beneficial results from their treatment in the homeopathic medical literature, however.[64]

One clinical trial has suggested homeopathic treatment to slightly reduce the adverse effects of radiation therapy in patients with breast cancer.[65]

Dosage and Toxicity:

Homeopathic medications can be given as a single dose or multiple doses taken over time. Adverse effects with homeopathic medicine are extremely rare. Because of the dilute nature of these remedies, adverse interactions between homeopathic medicine and conventional treatments are unlikely.

REVICI THERAPY

The Revici cancer therapy is a complex cancer treatment program that bears the name of its originator, Emanuel Revici (1896-1998). His treatment protocols were painstakingly described in his 1961 book.

Most of his treatments were believed to involve different combinations of minerals and fatty acids. He had an extensive battery of tests to determine how to tailor his treatment protocol for each individual.

Although Dr. Revici is no longer living, his Revici Life Science Center remains open in New York City.

Evidence:

As his treatments varied so widely from person to person, it is difficult to assess the potential validity of his treatment as a whole. While animal and *in vitro* research suggests that many different minerals[66,67] and fatty acids[68,69] may have anti cancer effects, it is not clear how applicable this research is to Revici's treatment.

A panel of New York physicians reviewed the results of Revici's treatment for two years. Their conclusion, published in 1965, was that none of the patients reviewed had any objective response to treatment.[70] Revici submitted a detailed rebuttal to this analysis, which was never published.

Dosage and Toxicity:

Because treatments are so individualized, dosages vary widely. Although high doses of minerals are used in some patients, and minerals can be very toxic in excessive amounts, no serious toxicity of Revici treatment has been reported.

LOW-SUGAR DIETS

Many popular books have advocated a low-sugar diet as an adjunctive treatment for patients with cancer. The popular notion is that sugar metabolically feeds the cancer, allowing it to grow faster than it would in the absence of sugar. Low-sugar diets are likely the most common dietary treatment for cancer in the United States.

Most non-diabetic patients, however, maintain a blood sugar at a fairly consistent level, even when consuming a diet high in sugary snacks. Also, many patients receiving chemotherapy or radiation are on steroid medications that adversely influence blood sugar.

Evidence:

A few studies have proposed some possible detrimental effects of sugar. The amount of sugar in a small glass of orange juice has been reported to cause significant suppression of one measure of immune system function for up to four hours.[71] Also, the insulin that humans secrete in response to eating sugar has been theorized to stimulate the growth of certain cancer types, including colon cancer, but this has not been proven.[72]

There are some studies that demonstrate an elevated risk of certain cancer types (specifically lung and colon cancer) in people with impaired blood sugar[73] or eating a diet high in sugar.[74,75] None of these studies concluded that changing the diet after diagnosis of cancer would be of benefit, however.

Surprisingly, there is little evidence regarding different diet types and cancer prognosis. Most of these studies, particularly those on breast and prostate cancer, have identified saturated fat, not sugar, as the dietary component most predictive of poor survival.[76,77] One study in a mouse breast cancer model suggested lower survival associated with diets high enough in sugar to adversely effect blood sugar.[78]

Some sources recommend restriction of dietary fruit as a source of sugar. Recent evidence, however, shows lower all-cause cancer mortality in frequent consumers of fruit.[79]

Dosage and Toxicity:

There is no known risk involved with reducing sugar in the diet. Patients wishing to adopt a low-sugar diet should be careful to maintain a diet that is sufficient in calories.

1 Neri B, de Leonardis V, Gemelli MT, et al. Melatonin as biological response modifier in cancer patients. Anticancer Research 1998; 18:1329-32.

2 Blask DE, Sauer LA, Dauchy RT. Melatonin as a chronobiotic/anticancer agent: cellular, biochemical and molecular mechanisms of action and their implications for circadian-based cancer therapy. Current Topics in Medical Chemistry 2002; 2:113-32.

3 Xiu SC, et al. Inhibition of androgen-sensitive LNCaP prostate cancer growth in vivo by melatonin: association of antiproliferative action of the pineal hormone with mt1 receptor protein expression. Prostate 2001; 46:52-61.

4 Futagami M, et al. Effects of melatonin in the proliferation and cis-diamminedichloroplatinum (CDDP) sensitivity of cultured human ovarian cancer cells. Gynecological Oncology 2001; 82:544-9.

5 Lissoni P, Barni S, Ardizzoia A, et al. A randomized study with the pineal hormone melatonin versus supportive care alone in patients with brain metastases due to solid neoplasms. Cancer 1994; 73:699-701.

6 Lissoni P, Paolorossi F, Tancini G, et al. Is there a role for melatonin in the treatment of neoplastic cachexia? European Journal of Cancer 1996; 32:1340-3.

7 Lissoni P, Barni S, Mandala M, et al. Decreased toxicity and increased efficacy of cancer chemotherapy using the pineal hormone melatonin in metastatic solid tumor patients with poor clinical status. European Journal of Cancer 1999; 35:1688-92.

8 Lissoni P, Paolorossi F, Ardizzoia A, et al. A randomized study of chemotherapy with cisplatin plus etoposide versus chemoendocrine therapy with cisplatin, etoposide and the pineal hormone melatonin as a first-line treatment of advanced non-small cell lung cancer patients in a poor clinical state. Journal of Pineal Research 1997; 23:15-19.

9 Lissoni P, Meregalli S, Nosetto L, et al. Increased survival time in brain glioblastomas by a radioneuroendocrine strategy with radiotherapy plus melatonin compared to radiotherapy alone. Oncology 1996; 53:43-6.

10 Lissoni P, et al. Anti-angiogenic activity of melatonin in advanced cancer patients. Neuroendocrinology Letters 2001; 22:45-7.

11 Lissoni P, et al. A phase II study of neuroimmunotherapy with subcutaneous low-dose IL-2 plus the pineal hormone melatonin in untreatable advanced hematologic malignancies. Anticancer Research 2000; 20:2103-5.

12 Burzynski SR. Antineoplastons: history of the research (I). Drugs Under Experimental and Clinical Research 1986; 12:S1-9.

13 Hashimoto K, Koga T, Shintomi Y, et al. The anticancer effect of antineoplaston A10 on human breast cancer serially transplanted to athymic mice. Nippon Gan Chiryo Gakkai Shi - Journal of Japan Society for Cancer Therapy 1990; 25:1-5.

14 Tsuda H. Inhibitory effect of antineoplaston A10 on breast cancer transplanted to athymic mice and human hepatocellular carcinoma cell lines. Members of Antineoplaston Study Group. Kurume Medical Journal 1990; 37:97-104.

15 Tsuda H, Iemura A, Sata M, et al. Inhibitory effect of antineoplaston A10 and AS2-1 on human hepatocellular carcinoma. Kurume Medical Journal 1996; 43:137-47.

16 Badria F, et al. Immune modulatory potentials of antineoplaston A10 in breast cancer patients. Cancer Letters 2000; 157:57-63

17 Liau MC, Szopa M, Burzynski B, Burzynski SR. Quantitative assay of plasma and urinary peptides as an aid for the evaluation of cancer patients undergoing antineoplaston therapy. Drugs Under Experimental and Clinical Research 1987; 13:61-70.

18 Buckner JC, Malkin MG, Reed E, et al. Phase II study of antineoplastons A10 (NSC 648539) and AS2-1 (NSC 620261) in patients with recurrent glioma. Mayo Clinic Proceedings 1999; 74:137-45.

19 Tsuda H, Sata M, Ijuunin H, et al. A novel strategy for remission induction and maintenance in cancer therapy. Oncology Reports 2002; 9:65-8.

20 Tsuda H, Sata M, Kumabe T, et al. Quick response of advanced cancer to chemoradiation therapy with antineoplastons. Oncology Reports 1998; 5:597-600.

21 Burzynski SR, Kubove E. Phase I clinical studies of antineoplaston A3 injections. Drugs Under Experimental and Clinical Research 1987; 13:37-43.

22 Burzynski SR. Treatment of bladder cancer with antineoplaston formulations. Advanced Experimental Clinical Chemotherapy 1988; 2:37-46.

[23] Burzynski SR. Antineoplaston A10. Drugs of the Future 1985; 10:103-5.

[24] Durie BG, Soehnlen B, Prudden JF. Antitumor activity of bovine cartilage extract (Catrix-S) in the human tumor stem cell assay. Journal of Biological Response Modifiers 1985; 4(6):590-5.

[25] McGuire TR, Kazakoff PW, Hoie EB, et al. Antiproliferative activity of shark cartilage with and without tumor necrosis factor-a in human umbilical vein endothelium. Pharmacotherapy 1996; 16(2):237-44.

[26] Suzuki F. Cartilage-derived growth factor and antitumor factor: Past, present and future studies. Biochemical and Biophysical Research Communications 1999; 259:1-7.

[27] Lee A, Langer R. Shark cartilage contains inhibitors of tumor angiogenesis. Science 1983; 221(4616):1185-7.

[28] Sheu JR, Fu CC, Tsai ML, et al. Effect of U-995, a potent shark cartilage-derived angiogenesis inhibitor, on anti-angiogenesis and anti-tumor activities. Anticancer Research 1998; 18:4435-42.

[29] Davis PF, He Y, Furneaux RH, et al. Inhibition of angiogenesis by oral ingestion of powdered shark cartilage in a rat model. Microvascular Research 1997; 54(2):178-82.

[30] Morris GM, Coderre JA, Micca PL, et al. Boron neutron capture therapy on the rat 9L gliosarcoma: Evaluation of the effects of shark cartilage. British Journal of Radiology 2000; 73:429-34.

[31] Horsman MR, Alsner J, Overgaard J. The effect of shark cartilage extracts on the growth and metastatic spread of the SCVII carcinoma. Acta Oncologica 1998; 37:441-5.

[32] Prudden JF. The treatment of human cancer with agents prepared from bovine cartilage. Journal of Biological Response Modifiers 1985; 4(6):551-84.

[33] Puccio C, et al. Treatment of metastatic renal cell carcinoma with Catrix. Proceedings of the Annual Meeting of the American Society of Clinical Oncology 1994; 13.

[34] Milner M. Follow-up of cancer patients using shark cartilage. Alternative Complementary Therapies 1996; 2:99-109.

[35] Romano CF, Lipton A, Harvey HA, et al. A phase II study of Catrix-S in solid tumors. Journal of Biological Response Modifiers 1985; 4(6):585-9.

[36] Miller DR, Anderson GT, Stark JJ, et al. Phase I/II trial of the safety and efficacy of shark cartilage in the treatment of advanced cancer. Journal of Clinical Oncology 1998; 16(11):3649-55.

[37] Lu C. University of Texas, MD Anderson Cancer Center: Phase III randomized study of induction platinum-based chemotherapy and radiotherapy with or without AE-941, a shark cartilage extract, in patients with stage IIIA or IIIB unresectable non-small cell lung cancer. MDA-ID-99303, active, 03/21/2000.

[38] Champagne P. Aeterna Laboratories, Inc.: Phase III randomized study of AE-941 (Neovastat; shark cartilage extract) in patients with metastatic renal cell carcinoma refractory to immunotherapy. AETERNA-AE-RC-99-02, active, 10/24/2000.

[39] Champagne P. Aeterna Laboratories, Inc.: Phase II study of AE-941 (Neovastat shark cartilage) in patients with early relapse or refractory multiple myeloma, AETERNA-AE-MM-00-02, active, 04/04/01.

[40] Loprinzi C. Mayo Clinic, Rochester, MN: Phase II randomized study of shark cartilage (Benefin) in patients with advanced colorectal or breast cancer, NCCTG-971151, active, 08-31/2001.

[41] Hildenbrand GL, Hildenbrand LC, Bradford K, et al. Five-year survival rates of melanoma patients treated by diet therapy after the manner of Gerson: a retrospective review. Alternative Therapies in Health and Medicine 1995; 1:29-37.

[42] Austin S, Dale EB, DeKadt S. Long-term follow-up of cancer patients using Contreras, Hoxsey, and Gerson therapies. Journal of Naturotherapy Medicine 1994; 5:74-6.

[43] Eisele JW, Reay DT. Deaths related to coffee enemas. Journal of the American Medical Association 1980; 244:1608-9.

[44] Margolin KA, Green MR. Polymicrobial enteric septicemia from coffee enemas. Western Journal of Medicine 1984; 140:460.

[45] Kushi LH, Cunningham JE, Hebert JR, et al. The macrobiotic diet in cancer. Journal of Nutrition 2001; 131:3056S-64S.

[46] Van Dusseldorp M, Schneede J, Refsum H, et al. Risk of persistent cobalamin deficiency in adolescents fed a macrobiotic diet in early life. American Journal of Clinical Nutrition 1999; 69:664-71.

[47] Weitzman S. Alternative nutritional cancer therapies. International Journal of Cancer (Supplement) 1998; 11:69-72.

48 Leipner J, Saller R. Systemic enzyme therapy in oncology. Effect and mode of action. Drugs 2000; 59:769-80.

49 Prasad KN, Cole WC, Kumar B, et al. Scientific rationale for using high-dose multiple micronutrients as an adjunct to standard and experimental cancer therapies. Journal of the American College of Nutrition 2001; 20:450S-63S.

50 Cassileth BR, Lusk EJ, Guerry D, et al. Survival and quality of life among patients receiving unproven as compared with conventional cancer therapy. New England Journal of Medicine 1991; 324:1180-5.

51 Stock CC, Martin DS, Sugiura K, et al. Antitumor tests of amygdalin in spontaneous animal tumor systems. Journal of Surgical Oncology 1978; 10:89-123.

52 Moertel CG, Fleming TR, Rubin J, et al. A clinical trial of amygdalin (Laetrile) in the treatment of human cancer. New England Journal of Medicine 1982; 306:201-6.

53 Morrone JA. Chemotherapy of inoperable cancer: preliminary report of 10 cases treated with laetrile. Journal of Experimental Medical Surgery 1962; 20:299-308.

54 Leipner J, Saller R. Systemic enzyme therapy in oncology. Effect and mode of action. Drugs 2000; 59:769-80.

55 Gonzalez NJ, Isaacs LL. Evaluation of pancreatic proteolytic enzyme treatment of adenocarcinoma of the pancreas, with nutrition and detoxification support. Nutrition and Cancer 1999; 33:117-24.

56 Kaegi E. Unconventional therapies for cancer: 4. hydrazine sulfate. Canadian Medical Association Journal 1998; 158:1327-30

57 Chlebowski RT, Bulcavage L, Grosvenor M, et al. Hydrazine sulfate in cancer patients with weight loss. A placebo-controlled clinical experience. Cancer 1987; 59:406-10.

58 Chlebowski RT, Bulcavage L, Grosvenor M, et al. Hydrazine sulfate influence on nutritional status and survival in non-small-cell lung cancer. Journal of Clinical Oncology 1990; 8:9-15.

59 Loprinzi CL, Kuross SA, O'Fallon JR, et al. Randomized placebo-controlled evaluation of hydrazine sulfate in patients with advanced colorectal cancer. Journal of Clinical Oncology 1994; 12:1121-5.

60 Loprinzi CL, Goldberg RM, Su JQ, et al. Placebo-controlled trial of hydrazine sulfate in patients with newly diagnosed non-small-cell lung cancer. Journal of Clinical Oncology 1994; 12:1126-9.

61 Filov VA, Gershanovich ML, Danova LA, et al. Experience of the treatment with sehydrin (hydrazine sulfate) in the advanced cancer patients. Investigational New Drugs 1995; 13:89-97.

62 Filov VA, Danova LA, Gershanovich ML, et al. The results of a clinical study of the preparation hydrazine sulfate. Voprosi Onkologii 1990; 36:721-6. [Russian]

63 Hainer MI, Tsai N, Komura ST, et al. Fatal hepatorenal failure associated with hydrazine sulfate. Annals of Internal Medicine 2000; 133:877-80.

64 Montfort H. A new homeopathic approach to neoplastic diseases: from cell destruction to carcinogen-induced apoptosis. British Journal of Homeopathy 2000; 89:78-83.

65 Balzarini A, Felisi E, Martini A, et al. Efficacy of homeopathic treatment of skin reactions during radiotherapy for breast cancer: a randomized, double-blind clinical trial. British Journal of Homeopathy 2000; 89:8-12.

66 Redman C, Scott JA, Baines AT, et al. Inhibitory effect of selenomethionine on the growth of three selected human tumor cell lines. Cancer Letters 1998; 125:103-10.

67 Liang JY, Liu YY, Zou J, et al. Inhibitory effect of zinc on human prostatic carcinoma cell growth. Prostate 1999; 40:200-7.

68 Whitehouse AS, Smith HJ, Drake JL, et al. Mechanism of attenuation of skeletal muscle protein catabolism in cancer cachexia by eicosapentaenoic acid. Cancer Research 2001; 61:3604-9.

69 Senzaki H, Iwamoto S, Ogura E, et al. Dietary effects of fatty acids on growth and metastasis of KPL-1 human breast cancer cells in vivo and in vitro. Anticancer Research 1998; 18:1621-7.

70 Lyall D, Schwartz M, Herter FP, et al. Treatment of cancer by the method of Revici. Journal of the American Medical Association 1965; 194:279-80.

71 Sanchez A, Reeser JL, Lau HS, et al. Role of sugars in human neutrophilic phagocytosis. American Journal of Clinical Nutrition 1973; 26:1180-4.

72 Giovannucci E. Insulin and colon cancer. Cancer Causes Control 1995; 6:164-79.

[73] Shaw JE, Hodge AM, de Courten M, et al. Isolated post-challenge hyperglycemia confirmed as a risk factor for mortality. Diabetologia 1999; 42:1050-4.

[74] De Stefani E, Deneo-Pellegrini H, Mendilaharsu M, et al. Dietary sugar and lung cancer: a case-control study in Uruguay. Nutrition and Cancer 1998; 31:132-7.

[75] Slattery ML, Benson J, Berry TD, et al. Dietary sugar and colon cancer. Cancer Epidemiology, Biomarkers and Prevention 1997; 6:677-85.

[76] Jain M, Miller AB, To T. Premorbid diet and the prognosis of women with breast cancer. Journal of the National Cancer Institute 1994; 86:1390-7.

[77] Meyer F, Bairati I, Shadmani R, et al. Dietary fat and prostate cancer survival. Cancer Causes Control 1999; 10:245-51.

[78] Santisteban GA, Ely JT, Hamel EE, et al. Glycemic modulation of tumor tolerance in a mouse model of breast cancer. Biochemical and Biophysical Research Communications 1985; 132:1174-9.

[79] Hertog MG, Bueno-de-Mesquita HB, Fehily AM, et al. Fruit and vegetable consumption and cancer mortality in the Caerphilly Study. Cancer Epidemiology, Biomarkers and Prevention 1996; 5:673-7.

Chapter Seven

Cancer Survivors Speak About Diet and Exercise

A diagnosis of cancer makes people think in new ways about a lot of subjects. Among those subjects are diet and exercise. Before cancer, they may have thought about food in terms of satisfying hunger, creating pleasure, or perhaps managing their weight. After diagnosis, the focus often becomes the place of diet and exercise among the many means of regaining health or preventing recurrence.

In the excerpts that follow, three cancer survivors share their thinking about diet and exercise in relation to their illness. The statements differ considerably. Two are taken from speeches, and one from the introduction to a cookbook, and each was written by an unique individual. But all three show us the intellect of a cancer survivor redefining the place of food and physical activity in his or her life.

Dr. William Fair was a surgeon who reconsidered cancer treatment after being diagnosed with colon cancer. Speaking at a conference on comprehensive cancer care in June 1998, he describes the goal of treatment as slowing the cancer, extending life and improving the quality of life. He then goes on to explain the role of nutrition, exercise, stress reduction and other complementary techniques in achieving those ends.

Diana Dyer is a registered dietitian and three time cancer survivor. She used her knowledge of nutrition to shape a diet for herself to help prevent recurrence. In her book, A Dietitian's Cancer Story, *she describes both the choices she made and the principle behind them. The excerpt included here is from a presentation she made at AICR's conference, "Nutrition After Cancer." In it she summarizes the thinking that went into her book.*

Finally, Michael Milken, a philanthropist and prostate cancer survivor, made radical changes in his diet after being diagnosed in 1993. In the introduction to the first of two Taste for Living *cookbooks he developed with Chef Beth Ginsberg, he talks about how he made the transition and carries the discussion one step further as he explores making his new diet delicious as well as healthy.*

William F. Fair, MD, talks about polytherapy for cancer survivors:

It was René Descartes in his meditation on the existence of God who made the argument for separation between the psyche and soma, the mind and body, the spirit and substance. That separation has been carried into Western medicine. We're always looking for the magic bullet. Western medicine is always looking for one thing. We want the one cure for cancer. We're going to change the altered P 53 gene and that's going to take care of everything. We're going to have one antibiotic, we're going to have one this or that.[1]

Eastern medicine takes more of a holistic approach – if you will, polytherapy. I don't know that much about Eastern medicine, but what I'm learning is that the approach in the Indian or Chinese tradition has always been to do things that will stimulate the entire energy or *chi* or *prana* of the body. It's not just looking for one thing. It's a recognition that chronic disease, be it cancer or some other disease, is a manifestation of a disturbance in the entire body, not just one gene that has gone wrong.

Techniques we're going to talk about today include nutrition, exercise, stress reduction, and so forth, as a surgeon sees them, and how they can relate to standard medicine. As I'll try to do throughout this talk, I'd like to blend some experimental data with clinical observations. In our own laboratory, we took human prostate cancer, put it in a nude mouse, and followed this tumor along. You can actually weigh the tumor. We can measure things like PSA. What we're able to show is that these animals were started on a high-fat diet similar to what the average American eats. The control animals were fed a lower fat diet. The tumors in the animals with a 20 percent or less fat diet don't disappear, but they basically don't grow, or grow very slowly. There's a marked difference in the overall growth of the tumors.

We know that from the time that prostate cancer starts in men, say in their 30s, until the time it becomes clinically obvious, if it does, is probably 20 to 30 years. If we could simply double the time that it takes until the cancer is clinically obvious (change that 30 years to 60 years), that would be tantamount to a cure in most men. Again, it gets back to the idea of thinking of cancer as a chronic disease rather than one that we have to bring out all the big guns to cure, regardless of the side effects.

How much fat should we recommend men allow themselves if they want to avoid or slow the growth of prostate cancer? Based on our experiments and some of the clinical studies that we've done with Dr. Wynder at the American Health Foundation and also with Dr. Ornish at UC San Francisco, we feel that 20 percent of total calories in the form of fat should be the absolute upper limit. This means that, figuring 9 kilocalories per gram, about 44 grams per day should be the upper limit of fat intake.

How do we do that? Avoid some of the foods the average American eats. A Jack in the Box cheeseburger would take care of one and a half days of fat. If you go up to a Quincy Steakhouse T-bone, you're up to almost four days of fat in one meal. What is surprising is some of the food products that we think would ordinarily have little fat in them. Nathan's Chicken Platter, for instance, has two and a half days of fat in one platter. Here's Little Caesar's veggie pizza. That's 47 grams of fat in one veggie pizza.

Looking at micronutrients, what can we tell folks with prostate cancer? The major interest is in vitamin A and prostate. In Finland they did a study on alpha-tocopherol, beta-carotene and cancer prevention. It was based on the observation that smokers had a decreased incidence of lung cancer if they took vitamin A supplements. There were 29,000 men in this study. What they showed was that in men who were smokers who were taking beta-carotene (the vitamin A supplement), there was actually an 18 percent increase in the incidence of lung cancer.

A secondary end point for this study was looking at some of the other cancers. There was a 32 percent decrease in the incidence of prostate cancer. This experiment with vitamin A has been duplicated in our laboratories. We compared animals being fed a 40 percent fat diet plus vitamin A with those on a 40 percent fat diet alone. Even though the animals are on a high-fat diet, the growth of this tumor was markedly inhibited in the presence of vitamin A compared to the animals not receiving vitamin A. Therefore I feel that vitamin A also plays a role in prostate cancer prevention.

A year or so ago, there was a lot of excitement because of an epidemiologic study at Harvard by Giovannucci and his colleagues showing that with increased tomato products there was a decreased incidence of prostate cancer. Lycopene was thought perhaps to be involved. Lycopene is an antioxidant, the most potent of the carotene family. It has been shown to inhibit proliferation in a number of cancer cell lines. In our studies, however, when we started the human prostate cancer in the nude mice, and fed the animals lycopene, not only weren't the tumors inhibited, they actually seemed to grow a little bit faster.

We could find no inhibition of this human tumor in animals receiving lycopene. This doesn't mean that lycopene is not involved. There are a number of types of lycopene. But it may be that there is something else in tomatoes. I think it's inappropriate to start telling your patients that they should be taking lycopene until we have better evidence. Tomato products may be of some value, but just isolating lycopene and taking it alone is the wrong way to go.

Let's look at some of the other things. Let's look at exercise. A study of 40,000 women was conducted, contrasting their activity and mortality rates. For the women who rarely or never exercised, the death rate was arbitrarily set at one. Women who exercise as little as four times a week for 30 minutes had a death rate that was one-half that of the women who never exercised.

Just to show you we're not sexist, I want to mention a study with men that was published this year in *The New England Journal of Medicine*. This was a very interesting study because there was a 12-year follow-up. Men were asked how much walking they did. Those who gave a history of walking less than a mile a day were contrasted with those who walked more than two miles a day. Twelve years later, the overall death rate was 50 percent less in the men who walked more than two miles a day. The cancer death rate was two-thirds less. If this were a new drug that somebody could make a lot of money out of, it would be on every television station and in every newspaper in the country. Because it's exercise, it's not publicized very much, but it's more profound than any drug that we have in terms of preventing cancer.

What about stress? Does stress cause cancer? We know stress can alter the immune function, and the immune system can regulate tumor growth. We also know that both the type and magnitude of immune changes can influence tumor growth or the ability to metastasize. A lot of these things are relatively new because we didn't have the molecular biology techniques to measure these responses until very recently.

A study that came out last December looked at 93 HIV positive men. They did not have clinical AIDS. It was a 42-month prospective study. The men had medical and psychological assessments every six months. What they found was significant. It is the first prospective study to focus on stress and cancer. They found that with a higher stress level there was increased disease progression. The men with the most severe stress level had four times the increase in conversion from HIV positive to clinical AIDS compared to those who did not. Again, this was a prospective study, not just looking back and saying stress may have a role here.

Moving on to some other things such as group support and spirituality, this morning several speakers have talked about social isolation. There have been 8 large-scale studies in a 15-year period with a wide geographical variation. In each of these studies there was a significant relationship between social isolation and disease, with a two- to five-fold increased risk of premature death in those who were socially isolated. Dr. Dean Ornish, in his most recent book, made this comment: "I'm not aware of any other factor in medicine – not diet, not smoking, not exercise, not stress, not genetics, not drugs, not surgery – that has such a major impact on our quality of life, incidence of illness, and premature death from all causes." He was speaking of love and intimacy.

A very interesting study, particularly to physicians, was made of Johns Hopkins medical students in the 1940s. These students were all male. They were given a questionnaire assessing their closeness to their parents. The researchers wanted to test the hypothesis that the quality of human relationships is a factor in the development of cancer later on. This study is ongoing, and it has been evaluated up to 50 years afterwards. It shows that the best predictor of cancer, decades later, up to five decades later, was the closeness of the father-son relationship in early life. This predictive power did not diminish over time. It was not explained by other factors, including smoking, drinking or radiation exposure.

It's not only related to humans. I could mention some relevant animal studies. In one such study, which appeared in *Science* in 1980, they were examining the effects of cholesterol on arteriosclerosis. In this study they had rabbits in a cage, and each of the rabbits got the same diet. When it came time to sacrifice the animals and look for plaque in the coronary arteries, they found an amazing thing. All of the animals in the top cages had severe plaque in the coronary arteries. When they got down to the lower cages, there was about 40 to 60 percent reduction. The question was why? A whole series of experiments later, it turns out that the lady who came in to feed these rabbits couldn't reach the top cages, so she just pushed the food into the cage. She would take out the ones she could reach on the lower levels, and pet them and play with them. It turned out that social interaction was the most significant factor in reducing the coronary artery plaque in animals. That finding correlates with what we saw in humans.

Moving on to things like symptom control – acupuncture. When I was in medical school, acupuncture was thought to be really hocus pocus. We now know – especially in the area of oncology – that nausea and vomiting can be effectively controlled by acupuncture. For years neurologists and neuroanatomists have looked at what effect acupuncture has on the nerves. We can't show any effect, but again the difference between pain and suffering is often not appreciated. Pain is a physical process, but suffering is the perception of that experience. It's not unrealistic to assume that acupuncture can have an effect without actually altering the nerve pathways but simply the perception of that experience. We'll find more and more roles for the use of acupuncture in the oncology patient.

Herbal therapy goes back to Old Testament times. This is a quote from Ezekiel: "And on the banks on both sides of the river there will grow all kinds of trees. Their fruit will be for food, and their leaves for healing." While it's a standard in traditional Chinese and some of the Oriental medicines, it's become lost in Western medicine. Yet just within the last few years, we've seen that benign prostatic hyperplasia responds very well to saw palmetto, and St. John's wort works for depression. Most recently, probably the most exciting thing we have in the chemical treatment of prostate cancer is PC-SPES. *(Editor's Note: As this book goes to press, PC-SPES has undergone a voluntary product recall. See the discussion of PC-SPES on page 98.)* It is a combination of eight herbs. It has an effect like a phytoestrogen. It inhibits bcl-2, which is helpful in causing the cells to undergo programmed cell death or apoptosis. There's scientific evidence now that herbal medicine really does have a role.

Aromatherapy. I'm going to wind up with a couple of cute studies that fascinate me. If you take a female rat and mix her with a male rat and the female gets pregnant, she will go on to deliver rat pups. Once the female becomes pregnant, if you take the male out of the cage, the pups will be reabsorbed. If you separate the pregnant female from the male by a wire cage, so they can see and smell each other, but they can't touch, the pregnancy will go on normally. If you put them in the same box, the female is pregnant, and you put a glass partition between them so they can see but they can't smell, the fetus is reabsorbed. How does that work? I have no idea.

Just this year there was a fascinating study published on pheromones. These are defined as airborne chemical signals that cannot be detected by normal smell. They are released into the environment and are thought to affect the physiology and behavior of other members of the species. Many women have observed that when they live together, in a boarding school, convent, or so forth, they tend to synchronize their menstrual cycles. This was a study to try to see whether this anecdotal observation was really true.

They took a group of donors, and they wore pads in the axilla for eight hours. They took these pads, cut them up and dropped them in some alcohol. They also measured evening urine samples for the luteinizing hormone which tells you the phase of ovulation the woman was in, basal body temperature and progesterone. They took these pads from the donors and cut them up. Then they took the pads and wiped them above the top lip of some women who agreed to serve as recipients. They couldn't smell anything.

They were able to show the presence of two pheromones, one that appeared to be present before ovulation and the other after the women ovulated. They could show that if the donor was in the preovulation phase of the cycle, it would decrease the cycle in the recipient, in other words, make their bodies try to catch up. The opposite was also true. If the donor was at the time of ovulation or after, the effect on the cycle of the recipient was to lengthen the cycle, lengthen it out to get them in sync. The timing of ovulation in the recipients was manipulated by these chemical signals that could not be appreciated. This is the first definitive evidence in humans that such a thing exists.

Here's another thing that intrigues me. It has nothing to do with oncology but it reflects something that Bernie Siegel mentioned. Let's say a pregnant sea turtle wanders up onto the beach and lays eggs. All those eggs have absolutely the same DNA in every single egg. Whether or not it's a male or a female depends on the temperature of the sand. The eggs that are near the top, and get more of the sun's exposure and have the warmer temperature, come out female. The ones on the bottom come out male. No one has any idea how that is explained. Sir Denis Burkitt, who is well known for his studies in Burkitt's lymphoma, has a saying I always liked: "Not everything that counts can be counted." I think this is another one of those examples.

In conclusion, what is the future of complementary medicine? We are going to see more of it for a variety of reasons – the ineffectiveness of current treatment has a role, but is not the major reason, as a recent study pointed out. As a surgeon, and we recognize that surgery still cures more cancer than radiation and chemotherapy combined, but the surgeon has to recognize that we use surgery as a last resort. John Hunter, who was probably the father of modern surgery, said this in the 18th century: "Surgery is like an armed savage, who attempts to get that by force which a civilized man would get by stratagem." He didn't say it in so many words, but think about the mind-body connection. If a civilized man can use other approaches to effect the same thing as surgery, that's the way we would go. This is not to say that I believe that mind-body approaches should replace surgery, but certainly they have value as an adjunct.

Diana Dyer, RD, explains how she developed a cancer-fighting diet:

I am a three-time cancer survivor. I went to my oncologist upon finishing chemotherapy after my most recent cancer diagnosis, and I asked him what I thought was a very simple question: What can I do to help myself? I have been through chemo. I have been through surgery. What is next?[2,3]

My main goal was to minimize my risk of recurrence. I was ready to really take on a new phase. I have to tell you I spent the five to six months that I was on chemo mostly eating whatever I could tolerate in order to take in the calories. When treatment was over, I began to wonder what I should be eating. I asked my oncologist. After some silence, my oncologist actually said, "Well, you can eat right and exercise." What does that really mean?

All that I knew in 1995, when I finished chemotherapy, were the very general guidelines from AICR that were probably 10 years old. I had already done all that and I wanted to know whether there was something more I could and should be doing. As a registered dietitian, I had to decide whether I believed the expression "you are what you eat" or thought it was just a marketing slogan. I went back to the medical, nutritional and scientific literature trying to understand what we know and what we do not know about nutrition and cancer survivorship.

I decided that we are what we eat, and that it can make a difference. I had to look at myself and admit that even a registered dietitian can make her diet healthier. I already had a healthy diet, but I wanted to go to an ultra-healthy diet. I wanted to choose foods that were going to do two things for me. First, I wanted everything going in my mouth to have some component that was going to reduce that cancer process if not help eliminate it; second, food had to nourish my body and soul.

I reviewed the scientific literature. I read every anti-cancer diet book available that claimed to include foods that a clinic recommended to reduce your risk for cancer or treat your cancer. I decided that because there was so much conflicting information available, clearly no one knew what the answer was. So, using the scientific literature, I developed my own action plan, which is what I am going to talk to you about.

The very first thing I did for my family and me was to take us off what I call "The Fast Food 'R Us" track. I went back to cooking. I, like nearly everybody else, had really fallen into this trap of relying on convenient processed foods. I also made a commitment to having my family eat together at least once each day. That was not easy, but I list this number one because it was the most important to me. My family probably was a psychosocial support group for me, the driving force that kept me going and enabled me to do everything else.

I increased my exercise; other speakers will give us information about the importance, particularly for breast cancer patients, of weight control and exercise. I also decided to eliminate or reduce alcohol intake. For breast cancer there clearly is a relationship with alcohol. We do not understand completely on a biochemical level why increased alcohol intake necessarily increases risk for breast cancer. There are a couple of working hypotheses. So, rather than having a glass of wine or a beer with dinner without even thinking about it, now I think about it and have one very occasionally.

The issue of fat is usually the first one to come up. Whatever type of cancer you have, everybody seems to have the idea that you have to reduce the fat in your diet. Well, more than just reducing fat in the diet, we understand now that it is probably more important to look at the type of fat in our diet, not just the total amount. Monounsaturated fats that come from olive oil and canola oil and the omega-3 fatty acids that come from fish, flax and some other legumes are important fats to have in the diet to reduce that cancer process. The animal or saturated fats, along with trans fats, or hydrogenated fats that are in our processed foods probably add to the cancer-progressing load in our body, and so those are important for me to remove from my diet. However, the load probably also depends on what you need in your diet for weight control in terms of fat calories, which is why it is important to get some nutritional advice from the registered dietitians at your cancer center.

The first question I remember asking one of my professional colleagues was "What is the minimum amount of fat that we can eat but still maximize the absorption of the fat-soluble molecules in our food that actually have anti-cancer activity?" Most of you have heard about fat-soluble vitamins - vitamin E, vitamin A. For our bodies to absorb those from either food or supplements, we need a little bit of fat in our diet. I did not want to make my diet so low in fat that it was not going to permit the maximal absorption of all of these cancer-fighting fat-soluble molecules called phytochemicals from plants. My colleague actually had some unpublished data and said that 16 percent to 18 percent is what we need, but the range is more like 15 percent to 20 percent. I have taken my fat intake down to roughly 20 percent to 25 percent. I threw away the corn oil and the Crisco in my pantry, and all I use now is canola oil or extra virgin olive oil. I had never even bought a bottle of olive oil before, so I completely changed how I am cooking. I also consume a small amount of fat with the fruits and vegetables that I have as between-meal snacks to maximize the absorption of the fat-soluble phytochemicals from these fruits and vegetables that are going to have anti-cancer activity in my body.

I realized that if I wanted the most anti-cancer activity from my food, my food was going to come from plants, and I have eliminated meats from my diet. We are talking red meat, poultry and pork. My family still eats meat but the amount that they eat is considerably less than what we ever ate previously.

Was I going to still consume dairy products? Just about every opinion exists about this question. There actually are good scientific data from population studies showing decreased risks of breast cancer and colon cancer, in particular, with increased consumption of dairy products. We do not understand what the biochemical mechanism for that is, and there are a lot of working hypotheses. I did not eliminate dairy products from my diet, and I consume one to two servings per day. I do consume only organic lowfat dairy products.

I still eat eggs, probably three to four per week. I buy eggs from chickens that have been fed special food that increases their amount of healthy fats - omega-3 fatty acids.

I really did not consume a lot of fish before this, but fish consumption can decrease your risk of cancer. Salmon, albacore tuna and rainbow trout have the highest level of omega-3 fatty acids. I wanted as much from my diet as possible of the molecules that would interrupt, thwart, or reverse this cancer process. So, I eat fish regularly and so does my family. We probably have salmon, tuna, or trout two to three times every week.

Recommendations about consuming 25 to 30 grams of dietary fiber per day are in every pamphlet you pick up. I realized that my intake was no different from the average American's intake, which was 10 to 12 grams. I went to my pantry and threw out my white rice and bought brown rice, threw out my white pasta and bought whole wheat pasta. My family complained that the pasta was too chewy, so I found a brand - Eden Foods - that actually has pasta that is 50 percent whole wheat flour and 50 percent white flour, just for people like me and my family who were not willing to chew their whole wheat pasta. I also am committed to having beans and legumes every day in some way, shape or form.

Here is my other rule: I have nine or more servings of fruits or vegetables every day. I had already done my "five a day," and it may have delayed the onset of my cancers or even enhanced their prognostic factors. These fruits and vegetables have a lot of anti-cancer bang for your buck. People have asked me whether or not they could have a quart of orange juice for their nine servings? My answer is that they really need to maximize their cancer-fighting activity from fruits and vegetables by having many colors - deeply dark colors of fruits and vegetables - every day. Even yesterday, which was a travel day, I had six servings of fruits and vegetables on the airplane. I had the vegetarian lunch, tomato juice instead of a Diet Coke, orange juice instead of another Diet Coke, and a 16-ounce bottle of carrot juice that I had brought with me. This takes planning; it does not happen by accident.

In addition to legumes, nuts and seeds frequently get overlooked; when people talk about plant-based diets, they often refer only to fruits, vegetables and whole grains. However, Brazil nuts are a source of selenium, an antioxidant that also seems to have a role in reducing cancer. Hazelnuts or filberts actually are a source of taxol, which is a chemotherapeutic agent that was previously thought to come only from the bark of the Pacific yew tree. Multiple molecules are in these fruits and vegetables and these nuts and seeds, which is why variety is so important.

Herbs and spices all contain molecules that have anti-cancer activity. Use them liberally. Especially if you are reducing fat in your diet, you need these for flavor.

I now consume flax instead of just wearing it. I consume one to two tablespoons of whole flax seeds every day for the plant source of omega-3 fatty acids and lignans, which also have anti-cancer activity.

I wash all my produce to minimize my intake of pesticides and to also reduce my chance of getting a food-borne illness. For everyone here with a suppressed immune system, avoiding food-borne illness is critical.

My beverage of choice, in addition to water, is green tea. I carry my own little container of green tea bags in my purse, and I can ask for hot water wherever I go. Scientists - chemists from Japan's equivalent of our National Cancer Institute - have said that even though green tea cannot prevent every cancer, it is the least expensive and most practical method for cancer prevention available for the general public. Two published studies that I am aware of actually show decreased risk of recurrence for breast cancer patients with increased consumption - three to five cups a day - of green tea.

What about soy? I am a post-menopausal breast cancer patient with an estrogen receptor-positive tumor. I have been on tamoxifen. I am right in the middle of this controversial question. There are actually two questions to ask: Is soy safe to eat? Is soy helpful to eat? The first question needs to be answered first. Can I eat soy without it potentially fueling my tumor? The molecule of interest in soy is an isoflavone called genistein that may have even been misnamed as a phytoestrogen, but the real concern is that that molecule could fuel an estrogen-positive tumor.

However, what is important to remember is that whole soy foods contain multiple molecules, all of which have anti-cancer activity, and many of those molecules fight cancer in different ways. What we have is synergy in a whole food—multiple molecules working together. Many studies in the literature show increased length of survival for Japanese women who have breast cancer. This observation proves nothing. It is just interesting data for me and it gives me a comfort zone that consuming soy in amounts probably equivalent to what Japanese women do after their cancer diagnosis is probably not harmful. But by no means do data prove that. However, two studies that I am aware of showed an improved outcome for animals with breast cancer that were given tamoxifen and soy foods. A couple of human studies show that eating soy foods shifts our estrogen metabolites to a higher level of the type that does not fuel tumors.

I do not know whether we should be eating soy. I can only tell you that I have been eating soy for the past six years without a recurrence of cancer. I consume one to three servings of whole soy foods a day. Most of the soy that I consume is typically found in a Japanese or Asian culture. I am not a research study - I am what they call an anecdotal report, or a case study. I was diagnosed with estrogen-positive Stage 3 breast cancer in 1995. I had a modified radical mastectomy with four and a half cycles of chemotherapy, no radiation therapy. I was on tamoxifen for a full five years. I have consumed soy throughout this entire period without a recurrence.

On my website (http://www.CancerRD.com) I have two weeks of menus with all the recipes for what my family eats. I do not spend three hours in the kitchen, and these are family tested, both in terms of consumption and preparation. In my book I have an entire section on how to eat out. Americans spend $1 billion every day eating out or on take-out food, and restaurants do not help us make healthy choices. AICR has also been addressing this problem, and they have wonderful materials to help you figure out how to eat out and still maintain a healthy diet.

I have a plan but very little clinical science to back it up. I have established an endowment at AICR specifically to fund research projects that will study nutritional strategies after a cancer diagnosis, either during treatment or recovery, to optimize our odds for long-term survival. The endowment is funded primarily from the proceeds of my book, *A Dietitian's Cancer Story*, which is my personal experience and my personal plan. Nutrition is just one component of a total recovery plan for cancer survivorship, and I discuss a holistic approach to cancer recovery in my book.

Bottom line - and the first recommendation from AICR: Choose a diet that is predominantly plant based: multiple fruits and vegetables, nuts and legumes, whole grains and minimally processed starchy staple foods. I cannot say enough about this. I have changed my diet for life, for my life.

Michael Milken describes how to eat for health and pleasure:

When your life is on the line, changing your diet can be easy. I know. When I was diagnosed with advanced prostate cancer in 1993 at the age of 46, I went from tuna melts and peanut butter to rice cakes and steamed broccoli overnight.[4]

It is important to note that research on the role of diet in the progression of cancer is not yet conclusive. Researchers believe that wide global variations in the incidence of cancer are in part explained by differences in diet. But scientists are just beginning to understand how molecules in food and vitamins affect our bodies' cells and energize our bodies to fight cancer.

After five years of interacting with many of the world's leading scientists studying nutrition, I am increasingly convinced that it's not just what we eat in the typical American diet that puts us at a higher risk for cancer. It's also what we don't eat that contributes to the high incidence of cancer in the United States: one in two American men and one in three American women are diagnosed with cancer in their lifetime.

Like many of the estimated 11 million Americans living with cancer, I decided not to wait for rock-solid scientific evidence before changing my diet. Often we see relationships – the link between smoking and lung cancer, for instance – before scientists can document the exact molecular mechanisms that occur. Most important, I recognized that there is no harm, and probably a great deal of good, in beginning to eat low-fat foods rich in nutrients absent from the typical American diet.

In January 1993 I had my first complete physical in two years. It was just a few weeks after one of my closest friends, Steve Ross, the chairman of Time Warner, had died of prostate cancer. Thinking of Steve, I asked my doctor to run a simple PSA test, one of the ways prostate cancer can be detected. He said I was too young to be tested.

"Humor me," I said.

And so I learned, in February 1993, that I had advanced prostate cancer. After consulting with researchers at a scientific conference in Houston and undergoing several weeks of additional tests, I discovered that my life expectancy was 12 to 18 months.

I decided to shift my energy and concentration into changing my lifestyle and diet and taking charge of my own illness. A month after my diagnosis, I established CaP CURE, the Association for the Cure of Cancer of the Prostate. With the support of thousands of people, it has become the largest private funder of prostate cancer research.

Since childhood, I had viewed life as a constant quest for knowledge. I set out to learn about Eastern medicine and ways to energize the world's greatest creation: the human body. It seemed clear that my health had suffered from all those years of eating fatty foods, all the meals eaten in haste and on the go, and more recently the stress from my legal problems.

My search for answers led to a meditation center in western Massachusetts that was based on the Ayurveda tradition of India. There Lori and I learned more about Eastern medicine, herbal cures and relaxation. We invited a doctor trained in both Western and Ayurveda medicine to move into our house for a few months. Early in the morning and late at night, we worked on breathing techniques, herbal therapy, meditation and yoga.

I learned how massage can activate the body's t-cells, which fight cancer, and how aromatherapy can energize the immune system. I rented a house at the beach and went for long walks. The smell of the seashore and the water brought back childhood memories of walks with my father at Lake Arrowhead in California.

Another benefit of the beach, I learned, was sunlight. Studies supported by CaP CURE show that sunlight and vitamin D help reduce the growth of prostate cancer. The studies also found a higher incidence of hormone-related cancers in northern Europe and the northern U.S. than in the southern parts of those continents. I thought back on all those long days in my windowless Wall Street office, and all those winter days I set off for work in darkness and returned in darkness. I had seen no more daylight than a hibernating bear.

After years of fielding a thousand calls a day, I turned off the phones in part of my house. And I changed how I ate. One Ayurveda teaching was "Better to eat a stone sitting down than a meal standing up." Similarly, rabbinical law cautions against eating while standing. For someone who had eaten 2,000 to 3,000 meals standing at his desk, this was another chilling thought.

I decided to drastically reduce the fat in my diet, to nine grams a day. I stopped eating meat, desserts and most dairy products. But that wasn't good enough. I found that even a single serving of "light" peanut butter exceeded my daily fat allowance. While I felt virtuous eating a mixed salad, I discovered that even a small amount of my favorite dressings put me way over the top. Even margarine that is 100 percent fat could legally be labeled "nonfat," so long as it contained less than one-half of one gram of fat per serving.

But cutting down on fat was not enough. Research supported by CaP CURE showed that soy protein could be a critical missing ingredient. I learned that Americans have a five times higher incidence of prostate cancer than people living in Asia and eating a traditional Asian diet. These diets are typically rich in soy protein, which contains a nutrient called genistein. This chemical has been found in laboratories to interfere with the growth of prostate cancer cells and to inhibit angiogenesis, the new blood vessel growth required for tumor cells to spread throughout the body. Genistein appears to help fight all hormonal cancers, including breast cancer. Soy had never been a staple of my diet, but now I substituted tofu or tempeh for meat, and I began mixing soy protein isolate powder with water or fruit juice.

But until I found Beth Ginsberg, eating was more of a burden than a pleasure. Beth made it her mission to incorporate the latest scientific knowledge in her adaptations of old, favorite recipes. Soon I was enjoying foods and flavors I had written off as long-lost memories. She turned my medicinal soy protein drinks into fruit smoothies that reminded me of the delicious Swiss orange-chip ice cream I would get at Swensen's Ice Cream in Berkeley. I could hardly guess that the drink was full of substances like limonene and geraniol, which have been shown to curtail tumor growth.

Even the hot dogs I had devoured as a college student made a comeback. Instead of red meat and who knows what else, these hot dogs are made of tofu. Beth even created a casserole using these hot dogs along with my beloved Philadelphia soft pretzels. Beth reviewed scientific studies while formulating her recipes. When research supported by CaP CURE found that beans and lentils help lower levels of hormones that indicate prostate cancer risk, Beth found delicious ways to introduce these foods into my diet. When scientists reported that a chemical called lycopene found in cooked tomatoes seems to produce a reduced risk of prostate cancer, Beth added tomato paste to many recipes. After research on garlic and other Allium vegetables indicated that they inhibit growth in a number of tumor cell lines, Beth increased the use of garlic as a seasoning. And finally, when scientists discovered that curcumin, which is found in cumin and is the yellow pigment found in turmeric, inhibits the development of certain cancers, Beth increased its use in chili and employed it for coloring in a sauce in her version of Eggs Benedict.

One day I decided to really put my new diet and Beth to the test. I invited some colleagues to lunch. They were as far removed from the vegetarian crowd as you could get, and I wanted to see how they would react to one of my typical meals. Beth served Reuben sandwiches, and afterwards I asked my guests what they thought they'd eaten. No one guessed that the cheese and Russian dressing were soy-based and the meat was actually tempeh. They all thought the sandwiches were delicious. I knew that if die-hard carnivores like these were convinced, we were on to something good.

I was highly motivated to change my diet because I believed it could mean the difference between life and death. But I wondered: How do we teach our children to make changes now?

One answer might lie with science. Both skeptics and young people, I feel certain, will increasingly become convinced of the value of nutrition as science unlocks the secrets of the human body. I am confident that biology and chemistry will drive the scientific breakthroughs of the 21st century, just as the 20th century was shaped by physics and remarkable advances in engineering, mechanization, data storage and telecommunications.

As previous generations envisioned the future through the science fiction of Jules Verne, and my generation glimpsed it through "Star Trek," the children of today are just beginning to imagine no less remarkable innovations in biology. I am sure the day will come when our grandchildren will be as flabbergasted at how naive we are about the relationship between food and the human body as we are by our own grandparents' unease with such modern contraptions as the laptop computer and the cell phone.

While there is no magic formula or secret cure, I know that good health requires healthy eating. Thanks to scientists all over the world and to Beth Ginsberg, I have learned to make practical use of the latest nutritional research without giving up the joy of eating.

[1] "Complementary Therapy is an Essential Part of Cancer Treatment" delivered at the Comprehensive Cancer Care Conference (June 13, 1998); see the website of the sponsoring organization, the Center for Mind-Body Medicine, www.cmbm.org.

[2] American Institute for Cancer Research. Nutrition after cancer: the role of diet in cancer survivorship 2002: 4-11.

[3] Dyer D. A dietitian's cancer story: information and inspiration for recovery and healing from a three-time cancer survivor. Swan Press 2002. For more information on Diana Dyer's unique approach to healthy living after cancer, visit her website at: www.CancerRD.com.

[4] Milken M. Introduction. Taste for living cookbook. The Association for the Cure of Cancer of the Prostate (CaP CURE) 1998. Reprinted with permission of Miavita Inc. See also the Taste for living world cookbook. CaP CURE 1999.

adjunctive   Term used to describe therapies or regimens that are added to – not used in place of – conventional medicine. *See also* **alternative, conventional.**

ALL   Acute lymphocytic leukemia, a malignant cancer of white blood cells called leukocytes. ALL is the most common form of leukemia in children.

alternative   Term generally used to describe therapies or regimens that are used in place of **conventional** medicine. Compare **adjunctive.**

AML   Acute myelogenous leukemia (also known as acute myeloid leukemia or acute nonlymphocytic leukemia), a blood cancer that develops in specific types of white blood cells (granulocytes or monocytes).

anecdotal evidence   Information that is based on **testimonials** and word-of-mouth instead of data published in **peer-reviewed** scientific literature or multiple observations.

angiogenesis   The growth of new blood vessels.

animal model   One method of **laboratory study** that allows scientists to observe how making highly specific changes affects a complex, living organism. Animal models are useful for testing promising theories, but there are significant physiological differences between humans and animals. Also called animal study, *in vivo* study.

antioxidants   Substances found in many vegetables and fruits that have been shown to protect the body from damage incurred by substances called **free radicals.** Some antioxidants are made by the body naturally.

apoptosis   Programmed cell death.

cachexia   State in which abnormal metabolism causes a degree of weight loss that cannot be attributed to decreased caloric intake alone. Weight loss may occur because the body is not able to utilize the nutrients from food properly.

case-control study   One kind of human study that compares the recollected diets and/or behaviors of subjects with cancer (cases) to the recollected diets and/or behaviors of subjects who do not have cancer (controls).

case history   *see* **case study**.

case series   A collection of **case studies**.

case study   A record of the relevant medical details surrounding the treatment of an individual with cancer. Also called a case history.

cell culture   One kind of **laboratory study** that allows scientists to observe how making highly specific changes affects the kind of cellular processes that can lead to cancer. Cell cultures can be used to discover possible **mechanisms** involved in diet-cancer associations. However, a mechanism that exists under tightly controlled laboratory conditions may not exist in humans. Also called test tube studies, cell studies, *in vitro* studies. Studies that involve groups of cells are called **tissue cultures** or tissue studies.

cell line   Term used in tissue culture to describe the series of cells that are grown from the initial specimen.

cell study   *see* **cell culture**.

chart review   An analysis of clinical data relating to a patient's case.

clinical study   One kind of human study that involves changing the diet and/or behavior of human subjects to see how such changes affect the real-world symptoms and progress of a disease. In a clinical study, researchers generally separate subjects into groups and make a specific kind of change (an **intervention**) to one group of subjects while leaving another, similar group (the **control group**) alone. *See* **placebo-controlled**.

cohort study   One purely observational method of human research that tracks diet and disease risk in a group of individuals over several years. Also called a prospective study.

control group   In **clinical studies,** the group of human subjects whose behavior and/or diet remains unchanged or who receive a placebo. (*See* **placebo-controlled**.) Data from the control group are compared to data from the **intervention group.**

conventional   Term used to describe standard medical theory and practice based on the analysis of empirical evidence. *See also* **adjunctive, alternative**.

dose-response effect   In **clinical studies,** a result indicating that a substance's degree of effect occurs in a measurable and consistent ratio with the amount of the substance that is administered.

efficacy State of exerting a definable and measurable influence.

epidemiology Branch of science that investigates disease risk in (often very large) human groups. Some epidemiological studies compare diets and disease rates of different nations or regions. Other kinds of epidemiological studies involve smaller groups of human subjects (*see* **case-control, cohort,** and **intervention** studies). Informally referred to as human studies.

estrogenic Term used to describe the influence of the estrogen hormone or estrogen-like substances. High levels of circulating estrogen have been linked to increased risk for certain **hormone-dependent cancers.**

free radicals Byproducts of normal metabolism that are highly reactive and capable of inflicting the kind of excessive damage to cells and to DNA that can lead to cancer. *See* **antioxidants.**

glioma Brain tumor.

hormonal blockade The use of drugs to inhibit certain hormonal functions.

hormone-dependent cancers Cancers such as those of the breast, ovary and prostate that have been linked to influence of certain hormones. *See* **estrogenic, phytoestrogens.**

human study *see* **epidemiology.**

in vitro **study** *see* **cell culture, tissue culture.**

in vivo **study** *see* **animal model.**

initiation First stage of the cancer process, which occurs when the cell is exposed to a cancer-causing compound, usually in steps and over many years. Followed by two other stages, **progression** and **promotion.**

intervention In **clinical studies,** the specific change in diet and/or behavior that is made to one group of human subjects. The presence of such an intervention (such as beta-carotene supplements or a low-fat dietary regimen) is what distinguishes clinical studies from human studies that rely solely on observation, like **case-control** and **cohort studies.**

intervention group   In **clinical studies,** the group of human subjects whose diet and/or behavior are changed.

isoflavones   Phytochemicals found in soybeans and soyfoods that seem to possess estrogenic functions in the body. Currently being widely studied for their possible role in the prevention of **hormone-dependent cancers.**

laboratory study   Research that investigates how specific changes influence anatomical or cellular systems. Laboratory studies do not involve human subjects (*see* **clinical study, epidemiology**) but do involve cell/tissue cultures (*in vitro* studies) or animal models (*in vivo* studies).

mechanism   Term used to describe any specific biochemical pathways that may be shown to play a role in a diet-cancer association. For example, certain substances in broccoli seem to "switch on" enzymes that help the body rid itself of carcinogens. This enzymatic pathway seems to be an important mechanism.

metastasis   Spread of cancer from one part of the body to another.

mucosa   Mucus tissue that lines the digestive tract.

multi-center clinical trial   A large human study that is conducted at many different locations (and even in different countries) simultaneously. Multi-center clinical studies allow for a large and varied group of subjects.

neurotoxicity   The state of being specifically poisonous to nerves and nerve tissue.

peer-review   Process by which research is analyzed in terms of its objectivity and adherence to accepted scientific methodology. Established medical journals subject all papers to peer-review before publishing them. Compare to **anecdotal evidence, testimonial.**

phytoestrogens   Substances in plants (such as **isoflavones** and lignans) that seem to act as weak forms of estrogen in the body. It is believed that phytoestrogens block the cellular receptors for estrogen and thus help to weaken that hormone's **estrogenic** effects on the body. Recently, some research has suggested that even the comparatively weak effects of phytoestrogens may pose their own risk.

placebo-controlled   A kind of **clinical study** that is designed so that the **control group** receives an inert substance (such as a sugar pill) while the **intervention group** receives a medically active substance. Such trials may be blind (the subjects do not know to which group they belong) or double-blind (both subjects and researchers do not know).

progression Final stage of the cancer process involving the increased growth of cancerous cells into an invasive tumor. Ultimately leads to metastasis. Progression is preceded by **initiation** and **promotion.**

promotion Second stage of the three-stage cancer process, preceded by **initiation** and followed by **progression.** During promotion, certain chemicals and biological conditions that do not possess cancer-causing activity on their own can greatly enhance the formation of tumors.

prospective study *see* **cohort study.**

proteolytic enzymes Enzymes that digest proteins.

quality of life scores Statistical method used in clinical studies to measure various aspects of a patient's condition. Can include data related to physiological and psychological factors.

retrospective analysis Statistical method used to combine data from previous studies.

test tube study *see* **cell culture, tissue culture**

testimonial Statement from an individual patient that is often used by practitioners/marketers to support the use of **alternative** treatments or regimens, especially where **peer-reviewed** scientific data is lacking.

tissue culture One kind of laboratory study that allows researchers to make very specific changes on a cellular level and observe how these changes affect live tissues that have been removed from the body. Tissue cultures allow scientists to uncover the possible reasons (mechanisms) that a specific substance or substances may raise or lower cancer risk. Also called tissue studies, test tube studies. Studies that involve smaller groups of cells are called cell studies or **cell cultures.**

tissue study *see* **tissue culture.**

toxicity The state of exerting toxic or poisonous effects.

About AICR

The American Institute for Cancer Research is the third largest cancer charity in the U.S. and focuses exclusively on the link between diet and cancer. The Institute provides a wide range of education programs that help millions of Americans learn to make changes for lower cancer risk.

AICR also supports innovative research in cancer prevention and treatment at universities, hospitals and research centers across the U.S. The Institute has provided more than $62 million in funding for research in diet, nutrition and cancer.

AICR is a member of the World Cancer Research Fund International.

Also available from AICR:

Nutrition After Cancer: The Role of Diet in Cancer Survivorship

Paperback, 62 pages
Price: $12

At AICR's landmark conference on diet and the cancer survivor, researchers and clinicians detailed what is known about eating and exercising to recover from cancer and to prevent its recurrence. This publication contains edited transcripts of ten talks delivered at this conference:

- *One of the nation's leading experts on soy evaluates current research on the hotly contested benefits of soy foods for cancer survivors.*
- *A dicussion of the possible anti-cancer effects of flaxseed and where it might fit into the survivor's diet.*
- *A registered dietitian and cancer survivor gives advice on evaluating nutrition and supplement claims.*
- *A translation of current knowledge into a daily regimen of diet and exercise for cancer survivors.*

A Dietitian's Cancer Story: Information and Inspiration for Recovery and Healing from a 3-Time Cancer Survivor

Available in English and Spanish
Author: Diana Dyer, M.S., R.D.
Paperback, 112 pages
Price: $12

Diana Dyer survived neuroblastoma as a child and two separate breast cancers in adulthood. Now healthy and cancer-free, Dyer has turned her own survival story into a vehicle for educating others.

A Dietitian's Cancer Story is a useful guide for health professionals as well as cancer survivors. It discusses the nutritional components of Dyer's program, describes a "decision tree" for evaluating alternative and complementary therapies, and offers practical advice from her experience as both dietitian and patient. This inspiring book has been used by thousands of cancer survivors as they search for strategies to extend and improve their quality of life.

Proceeds from this book will be donated to the Diana Dyer Cancer Survivors' Nutrition Research Endowment at AICR.

To order call 1-800-843-8114 or go to www.aicr.org

American
Institute for
Cancer
Research